Coping With Difficult People
in the Health Care Setting

D0062064

 Practical Laboratory Management Series

The Practical Laboratory Management Series

Coping With Difficult People

in the Health Care Setting

William O. Umiker, MD
Adjunct Professor of Clinical Pathology
Hershey Medical Center
Penn State University
Hershey, Pennsylvania

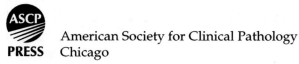
American Society for Clinical Pathology
Chicago

RA
971.35
.U525
1994

Publishing Team
Andrea Blumenfeld (layout/production)
Karen D. Johnson (editorial)
Renee Kastar (marketing)
Denise St. John (marketing)
Joshua Weikersheimer (publishing direction)

Printed on Recycled Paper

Library of Congress Cataloging-in-Publication Data

Umiker, William O.
    Coping with difficult people in the health care setting / by William O.
Umiker.
        p. 277   cm. — (Practical laboratory management series)
    Includes bibliographical references and index.
    ISBN 0-89189-361-X
    1. Health facilities—Personnel management. 2. Medical personnel—Job
stress—Prevention. 3. Communication in personnel management. 4. Problem
employees. 5. Interpersonal relations. 6. Interpersonal conflict. I. Title.
II. Series.
    [DNLM: 1. Interpersonal Relations. 2. Communication. 3. Personnel
Management—methods. 4. Health Facilities—organization & administration.
WX 159 U485h 1993]
RA971.35.U525 1993
362. 1'1'0683—dc20
DNLM/DLC   93-1079
for Library of Congress   CIP

Copyright © 1994 by the American Society of Clinical Pathologists. All rights
reserved. No part of this publication may be reproduced, stored in a retrieval system,
or transmitted in any form or by any means, electronic, mechanical, photocopying,
recording, or otherwise, without the prior written permission of the publisher.
Printed in the United States of America.

06 05 04 03 02 6 5 4 3 2

Contents

Preface

A decade ago, I had the good fortune to read Dr. Robert M. Bramson's book, *Coping With Difficult People*, and subsequently listen to his audiotapes. What impressed me the most were his revelations regarding the psychosocial pathogenesis of the various forms of annoying folks. He combined this with practical advice on how to deal with each of the aberrant behavioral types. Subsequently, I used much of what I learned from Dr. Bramson when confronting the problem people encountered in the practice of laboratory medicine—his techniques work! When I retired from my administrative duties to become a writer and lecturer, I found that my audiences were also fascinated with Dr. Bramson's teachings.

Many books have been published on this topic since Bramson's made the scene. Bramson and others focused on reactive remedies, principally confrontational skills. As a physician, I prefer preventive measures—proactive strategies that can prevent the development of problem employees or abort minor behavioral problems before they become disruptive. That is what I attempt to do in this book. This information is vital to hospital and laboratory managers when dealing with difficult employees, customers, and patients. My approach is unique in that I focus on the personnel problems specific to these health care professionals. I have adapted the coping techniques to address the particular demands of this work environment and the usual people problems that result.

This book is structured to teach you the principles, from basic concepts to specific examples, for dealing with difficult people. The essential skills of communications, assertiveness, and stress resistance are emphasized throughout. You will learn the management techniques for hiring, training, coaching, counseling, and disciplining employees. Then, we will delve into the various categories of difficult folk, from underperformers to chronic complainers, from hostiles to sexual harassers. Along the way, we will reinforce the proactive coping strategies necessary to keep these difficult people under control.

Finally, this text employs a somewhat unique editorial convention for handling the issue of gender. Since both supervisors and employees can be either male or female, we have varied the gender of the personal pronoun used in each chapter. Therefore, "the boss" may be a she in chapter 6 but shift to a he in chapter 11. The change not does indicate specifics but only provides for variety.

Acknowledgments

As noted in the Preface, I am greatly indebted to Dr. Robert Bramson for his inspirational leadership in focusing on difficult people at work and for granting me permission to use his terminology.

Without the encouragement and support of Joshua Weikersheimer, Director of ASCP Press, this book would not have been so readily available to laboratory workers and other health care providers. Joshua has been a patient and caring mentor.

Karen D. Johnson, my editor, has been a gem. I have dealt with other competent editors, but Karen is in a class by herself. She proved to be an interested reader as well as an editor, and she made many helpful suggestions for improving content as well as readability.

My library research was made easy through the cooperation of Pat Buch Miller and her staff. They responded to all my requests with enthusiasm and quickness.

I am beholden to all the difficult people in my life who provided me with opportunities to study their idiosyncrasies and to practice my limited interpersonal skills. In retrospect, there were not that many of them, and this forced me to learn about many of these challenging individuals from the experience of other writers and seminar leaders.

Finally, I must thank my wife, Nora, who spends many dull evenings at home because my writings and seminars often have a higher priority than does our social or family activities.

1. Let's Meet These Difficult People

Difficult people come in a bewildering array of characters—no two are exactly alike. Whatever their particular idiosyncrasies or problems, most of them display some or all of the following characteristics described by Tucker.[1]

- Their annoying behavior is repetitious.
- We think of them often, at work and at home. Our spouses know them well, even though they have never met.
- We get tense when we see them coming or even hear their names.
- We wonder how much longer we can take it.
- We avoid them as much as possible. They make us want to stay home instead of going to work.
- Our "common sense" coping methods have failed.

While each of us may occasionally annoy one of our fellow human beings, a difficult person's unpleasant behavior is habitual and affects most of the people with whom he comes in contact.

WHY IT IS DIFFICULT TO COPE WITH DIFFICULT PEOPLE

Most managers agree that dealing with problem people—or, people with problems—is their most challenging responsibility. At least three factors make this challenging:

1

1. Difficult people rarely feel that they are difficult or in need of help.[2]
2. If we were honest with ourselves, we would admit that we wished these people were more like us. Therefore, our intuitive inclination is to try to restructure their personalities or attitudes. Such efforts are doomed to failure!
3. The behavior that we find so annoying has apparently served these people well—at least they think that it has.

To achieve a significant behavioral modification, we must convince these individuals that they indeed have a problem and that a change is in their own best interest.

DEFINITION OF COPING

Formal definitions of the verb "to cope" include: "to contend with," "to pit oneself against," and "to struggle with." These definitions suggest that trying to cope with difficult people is just that—difficult! Substituting "challenging" for "difficult" is a change in semantics that does not make our task any easier.[2]

Coping strategies can be reactive or proactive. Reactive strategies attempt to minimize the impact of other people's difficult behavior, but they do not address the real sources of the problem. These techniques help us to "get through" difficult situations but do not really solve the long-term issues. Proactive strategies, on the other hand, strive to prevent people problems from developing. If problems do occur, proactive managers deal with them immediately before they explode into major problems. Thus, proactive techniques are more effective in the long run than merely reactive "bandaid" solutions. Throughout the text, I will emphasize the less stressful and more efficient proactive approach to confronting difficult people.

Both of these forms of coping provide an alternative to acceptance of the other person's behavior or to futile attempts to change the person. Although acceptance avoids the immediate unpleasantness of confrontation, it reinforces the undesirable behavior. As Bramson[3] notes, "Trying to change another person's personality can be the world's greatest hard luck story."

DIFFICULT EMPLOYEES WILL BE EMPHASIZED

Employees who are satisfied with their working conditions and relationships are more likely to pass these good feelings along to their customers. If the needs and wants of patients, clinicians, and other recipients of health care services are to be met, administrators must first achieve employee satisfaction and eliminate the adverse impact of problem employees. These managers must also be trained to cope with problem customers and coworkers. Thus, by learning the management skills necessary for coping with difficult employees, the prevailing goal of providing better customer services can be achieved.

THE HEALTH CARE ENVIRONMENT IS UNIQUE

This text focuses on the specific personnel problems encountered in the health care industry. The people and the situations found in medical laboratories and hospital/nursing facilities differ from those one meets in other work environments. Every hospital has two organizations under the same roof: a hospital hierarchy and a medical staff, each with its own leaders and regulations or bylaws. A recent evolution of hospital middle management has witnessed increased shared governance. Many departments have both a technical or administrative director and a medical or professional director. Dual roles such as these can increase the possibility of conflicts and divergent goals. As medical technologists and nurses struggle to achieve a professional status comparable to that of pathologists and physicians, new clashes are erupting.

Managers who move into health care institutions from nonmedical organizations frequently observe that dealing with health care professionals and technical specialists is not always easy. These medical people often have more loyalty toward their profession or specialty than they have toward their employers. Because of the demands of their work environment, they often feel that they should be exempt from some of the policies and procedures that other employees must follow. Because of the vital nature of the work performed, they may expect special treatment. Thus, managing these people demands special expertise. Past tolerances of idiosyncrasies are rapidly disappearing as medical caregivers struggle to be more consumer-oriented and cost-effective.

Additionally, modern-day patients bring a special set of challenges to caregivers. They are more knowledgeable about medical care than their predecessors, more demanding, more critical, and more litigious—great opportunities for conflict and emotional upsets.

The organizational changes in the health care industry pose additional challenges for managers and employees. The bottom line is providing the highest quality of customer services possible. The ability to handle the difficult problems and deal with the difficult people you are liable to confront will often be the key to your success. We hope this text will help you achieve that goal.

REFERENCES

1. Tucker RK. *Fighting It Out With Difficult People*. Dubuque, Iowa: Kendall Hunt Publishers; 1987.
2. Keating CJ. *Dealing With Difficult People: How You Can Come Out on Top in Personality Conflicts*. Ramsey, NJ: Paulist Press; 1984.
3. Bramson R. *Coping With Difficult People*. New York, NY: Anchor Press/DoubleDay; 1981.

2. Powerful Communication Skills

Any company in search of excellence has only two basic places to look: at the quality of its people and the quality of the way its people communicate."[1]

Poor communication can lead to conflict and unhappy relationships at work. On the other hand, powerful communication strategies often provide the key to prevention and resolution of personnel problems. Good communication depends not just on clear pronunciation, a careful choice of words, and a smiling face; rather, it stems from a feeling of rapport—the key to conscious contact. Managers must be authentic and acknowledge people's feelings, which provides the empathy so vital in communications. Acknowledging feelings does not necessarily mean agreement, but only a willingness to listen to expressions of these emotions and to indicate that it is acceptable to have such feelings.

KEEPING THE LINES OF COMMUNICATION OPEN

Successful communication also includes keeping employees, bosses, and coworkers apprised of information they need to know. Many employees feel that their leaders hold back things that they should be told. Every time a manager comes back from a meeting with the top brass or a senior executive comes out of a supervisor's office, the staff's interest is piqued. Likewise, subordinates may withhold important information from their superiors if they dislike or mistrust them or if they fear that the information will adversely affect their relationship. Such communication blocks impede the development of a productive work atmosphere.

BARRIERS TO COMMUNICATION

There are three major categories of communication barriers: physical, semantic, and psychological. Physical barriers include background noise, visual distractions, poor lighting, and environmental discomforts such as excessive heat or cold. The most obvious semantic barriers are language differences; but jargon, computerese, acronyms, and professional terminology can be just as confusing.

Physical and semantic barriers are often easier to overcome than psychological barriers. Potential psychological barriers include perceptions, values, and assumptions. Perception is knowledge obtained through experience or intuition. For example, two people witnessing the same scene or listening to the same speech may perceive entirely different messages based on their perceptions. We tend to see what we are looking for or what we expect based largely on our individual past experiences. Values are what we were taught to believe. Cultural, racial, and gender differences impact our value systems. Initially, the amount and kind of educational and religious training we receive formulate our value systems. These are modified by our social and financial status and by daily multimedia exposure. Values have a major impact on the type of dialogue that takes place in any given situation. To learn more about the value systems of others and ourselves, listen for the "should's" and "should not's" in people's language: "Promotions should be based on loyalty and length of service"; "Supervisors should not tell us how we must dress."

Assumptions are cognitive things taken for granted—how people think things are. Frequently assumptions turn out to be false or distorted. A manager hears laughter in the next room and assumes that the employees are goofing off or are poking fun at her. When we teach or direct we may ask "Do you understand?" and "Do you have any questions." We assume that a "yes" to the first question and a "no" to the second indicates that our message was understood, but we really do not know without testing that knowledge. Students and employees are often reluctant to admit that they did not understand the message, or they may think they understand but they really do not. Assumptions are also complicated by nonspecific messages (eg, "Will you make me a few copies?" or "Please finish that report as soon as possible").

Other psychological barriers include inconsistencies between words and facial expressions, voice tone and body language; distinguishing kidding from sarcasm; put-downs ("Do not be ridiculous..."); judgmental responses ("The trouble with you is..."); stereotyping ("You women just do not understand instrumentation..."); and inflammatory utterances ("I demand that you...").

These communications barriers cannot be completely eliminated. The goal of effective communications, however, is to be more aware of these potential barriers and to work toward overcoming them.

AUDITORY COMMUNICATION: LISTENING

Failure to listen not only has an adverse effect on employee relationships, it also affects the quality of care given to patients. For example, a patient's complaints may be overlooked or the patient may feel that she is being neglected. Most of us are poor listeners. We talk when we should be paying attention to others. Even when we are not talking, we are often merely waiting to speak rather than listening. We are often guilty of mentally writing a script—formulating a response while the other person is still verbalizing.

How one says something is just as important as what that person says. Voice tone, volume, and rate vary with one's emotional state.[2] For example, a subordinate may say "I am okay," but her delivery of the message reveals "I feel miserable."

VISUAL COMMUNICATION: BODY LANGUAGE

"Listening" is visual as well as auditory. In fact, when what we "see" is different from what we "hear," the visual messages are usually the genuine ones. Here are some commonly observed visual messages:

> Clearing throat, blinking eyes = "I am nervous."
> Tugging on ear = "I am not listening."
> Rubbing nose = "I do not believe that."
> Clasping hands behind head = "I am in charge here."
> Rubbing palms = "Let's go" or "I am winning."
> Arms folded across chest = "The answer is no."
> Rubbing back of neck = "I am frustrated."
> Moving foot in circle = "I am getting impatient."
> Raising one eyebrow = "I cannot believe this."
> Raising both eyebrows = "That surprises me."

KINESTHETIC COMMUNICATION: TOUCHING

Touching complements verbal messages but must be done in a way that is not interpreted as having sexual or aggressive overtones. Important factors in the appropriate use of touching are the location, the kind, and the context. Safest touch zones are the forearm, elbow, upper arm, and shoulder.

Use light, transient touches. Do not hold, pat, or massage. Handshakes are almost always appreciated except when they produce pain (people with arthritis dread them) or when they are too prolonged.

The context of the conversation often determines the appropriateness of using touching as a communication method. The touch should reinforce the verbal response. It is especially appropriate when expressing appreciation or support.

When you receive an unwelcome touch, say how you feel about it. Be explicit (eg, "Dr. Smith, when you put your arm around my shoulders like that, it makes me uncomfortable. Please stop it"). We will get into the problem of sexual harassment in greater depth in chapter 25.

NEUROLINGUISTIC PROGRAMMING

Researchers Bandler and Grinder[3] developed a theory known as neurolinguistic programming (NLP). According to this theory, individuals perceive their environment mainly in one of three representational systems: visual, auditory, or kinesthetic.

Visualizers think in terms of images and are more sensitive to their visual surroundings. These people use words such as see, look, show, focus, image, perspective, or picture (eg, "I see what you mean").

Auditorily oriented individuals are more sensitive to what they hear. They focus on words, voices, and other sounds. Their favorite words are hear, sound, articulate, enunciate, verbalize, or express (eg, "That new policy sounds unfair to me").

People in the kinesthetic group perceive the world through emotional and tactile feelings. They recall events in terms of how or what they felt. They frequently use these words: grasp, feel, smooth, rough, and handle (eg, "I feel that you are making a big mistake").

NLP appears to be of practical value. Many organizations have hired NLP experts to teach the theory to their employees. Communication is apparently improved when you match the listener's proclivity with the congruent words. Alert instructors use NLP to tailor their teaching methods to trainees. The instructors will use manuals, visual aids, computer printouts, and written reports for the visualizers. Instruction of the auditorily oriented students will feature tapes, lectures, and other verbal instruction. The kinesthetics prefer hands-on training.

THE VALUE OF SILENT PAUSES

Pausing is a great way to get people to speak up and to reveal what is on their minds.[2] This technique is very effective when sensitive topics come up during interviews or counseling sessions—when the other person stops talking and appears hesitant. Lean forward and look as though you expect her to say something more. Slowly and silently count to ten before you break the silence. Usually the person will speak up before that time has elapsed.

Shorter pauses are also recommended. They provide opportunities to reflect on the context of the communication before responding and reduce the likelihood that you will say something you regret later. If you are not listening well and you start to talk when a person pauses between sentences to catch her breath, you are interrupting, which is indicative of nonlistening or impoliteness. A tendency to finish people's sentences is equally bad.

AVOID VERBAL PATTERNS THAT REDUCE POWER

The following verbal patterns should be avoided. Because these tactics are indirect, they reduce the power of the message you are trying to communicate.

1. Posing questions to make requests or demands: "Would you like to place this sample in the specimen refrigerator?" Instead say, "Please place this sample in the specimen refrigerator."
2. Using disclaimers: "I know this sounds silly, but...." Instead, simply say what is on your mind.
3. Using weak qualifiers: "sort of," "maybe," "a little bit." Eliminate these from your vocabulary.
4. Tolerating interruptions: Do say, "Leon, I was not quite finished." Then go on.

The best way to communicate is the most direct and straightforward way.

THE THREE STRATEGIES FOR EFFECTIVE COMMUNICATING

"Seek first to understand—then work to be understood."[4] To make sure the message is received, a good listener must employ all three of the following communications strategies.

Attentive Appearance

Attentive appearance includes the appropriate position, eye contact, facial expression, and body language. Position yourself facing the person and honor her personal space (usually 3 to 4 feet). Stand or sit upright. Look relaxed and interested. Do not position furniture between you and the other person (this includes your desk).

When two people like one another, they establish eye contact more often and for longer duration than when there is dislike or tension in the relationship.[5] Good eye contact is not staring down the other person ("reptile stare" or "soldier stare"). Rather, it is achieved by focusing on another part of the person's face, shifting one's gaze from the eyes to the nose or other parts of the face, and occasionally glancing away from the face entirely.

Appropriate facial expressions include frowns, smiles, and raised eyebrows, with headshakes and nods as appropriate. Your body language must be congruent with the verbal message you are sending. For example, your arms crossed in front of your chest suggests that you are not open to new ideas.

All this attentiveness looks good, but the sender is still not certain that the message has been received and understood.

Attentive Words

Attentive words include phrases such as: "Uh-huh," "Yes, go on," "I see," "Oh?" "Tell me more," and "How did you feel at that point?"

This sounds good, but the sender is still not certain that the message is getting through.

Feedback

Feedback includes paraphrasing and interpreting what the other person is saying, so she knows that you are listening.

Paraphrase: "First, I pick up the report in the office"; "At that point you were pleased."

Interpret: "What I hear you saying is…"; "Do you mean that…?"; "You are saying…right?"

Now the sender knows that the message has been received and is understood. Feedback is the most important strategy.

KINDS OF RESPONSES

- Defensive: "That is a lie."
- Judgmental: "You are too sensitive."
- Advisory: "I will tell you what I would do."

- Questioning: "Be more specific."
- Empathetic: "You seem upset—I can understand that."

Skilled listeners make use of empathetic or supportive responses, and minimize defensive, judgmental, and advisory responses. Questioning is good unless it sounds like cross-examining.

AVOID THIS BAKER'S DOZEN

- Advising
- Criticizing
- Cross-examining
- Diagnosing
- Diverting
- False praising
- Feigning listening
- Insincere reassuring
- Moralizing
- Name calling
- Ordering
- Threatening
- Using logic with a distraught person

FIVE GREAT TIPS FOR BETTER COMMUNICATION

1. Devise an "open door policy," so that employees know that you are available whenever they need your advice or counsel. Implement this policy in locations other than your office. Be available in the lounge during breaks or in the dining room at meal times. Some people, especially small groups, are more comfortable talking to you there rather than in your office.

2. Be honest about your biases.[2] It is okay to admit that you hold a certain point of view about an issue.

3. Listen for underlying feelings. Pay attention to body language, voice tone, inflections, and repetitious words. When an employee complains about laboratory personnel not getting any recognition, she may be saying that you are not paying enough attention to her.

4. Never say "You are wrong." If you must dispute what a person says—especially if the other person is a know-it-all or your boss—say something like "What you say seems to make sense. How would you answer someone who argues that...?"

This is known as the "strawperson" technique because it diverts attention away from you and gives you an opportunity to back down or to escape direct attacks.

5. Respond to suggestions by using the PIC technique:

P = Positive. Say something positive about the suggestion if you approve: "Good idea. How can I help?"

I = Interesting. Ask for more information: "That sounds interesting. Tell me more."

C = Concern. Instead of a negative remark, be tentative: "I have a problem with that idea. How would you...?"

HOW TO GIVE AND TAKE NEGATIVE FEEDBACK

Criticism is frequently involved when dealing with difficult people. Criticizing is a part of your responsibility as a coach. It is the core aspect of counseling and disciplinary meetings. This core can undergo a tragic meltdown when the criticism is excessive or when it is not balanced by positive stroking. When subordinates are under fire they often become defensive and counterattack. Therefore, it is essential that you can take it as well as dish it out.

When You Are Dishing it Out

Your goal in criticizing is to alter behavior, not to castigate the person. Here are some practical suggestions:

1. Do not attempt to soften the blow to the person's self-esteem by sandwiching criticism between slices of irrelevant praise. The recipient will either be confused or will feel manipulated. But, do link positive and negative comments when the connection is relevant. For example, "Rita, you almost always get to work on time—I appreciate that. Do you think that you could be equally prompt with your monthly report?"
2. Criticize as soon as possible after the act, but not before you have the necessary information.
3. Avoid criticizing when you or the other person is emotionally upset.
4. Make the criticism a dialogue between two adults, not a parent/child transaction. Do not scold or belittle.
5. Avoid absolute terms such as "always" or "never" (eg, "You are always late").

6. Be specific or give examples. Change "You never consider other people's feelings," to "Three times this week I heard Louise break into tears when you yelled at her."
7. Give the person time to respond and then listen intently to her reply.
8. Avoid expressing a demand as a "Why." For example, "Why do you keep interrupting me?" Do you really expect an answer? Instead say, "Please stop interrupting me."
9. Substitute "and" for "but." A "but" invalidates everything that precedes it, while an "and" validates it. For example, "Your work has improved, but..." is better expressed as "Your work has improved, and if you can..., I think there will be still more progress."
10. How you say something and the accompanying body language you use often determine whether or not you get the behavior you seek. For example, if you say, "Frank, be more careful how you talk to callers" in a whining, exasperated tone, the message you send is that you really do not expect Frank to comply with that request.
11. Explain why behavioral change is needed. For example, when you advise, "Do not hang up the phone until you know the call has been transferred," add this additional comment, "otherwise some callers will not reach their party."

When You Are Taking it

Your goal in receiving criticism is to benefit from it, not to overcome the critic. This requires that you switch from an emotional response to a cognitive one. Do not take the comments personally, but concentrate on the behavior that is being criticized. Here are some practical suggestions:

1. Accept the criticism as a mature person. Do not deny, become defensive, or counterattack. Do not stonewall or make excuses: "That is not in my position description," or "We were very busy and understaffed."
2. Do not retaliate or accept criticism only superficially: "You should talk. How about the time that...?" or "Okay, okay, big deal" (said sarcastically).
3. Take notes. It shows that you have sincere interest and also helps to keep you from making an emotional response.
4. If the critic complains about subjective factors such as attitude or professionalism, insist on examples.
5. Make sure that you understand the criticism by paraphrasing what was said.
6. Probe for more specific information. This negative inquiry encourages the critic to be more objective. For example:

You: "I understand that you complained to my boss about my work. Please tell me what was wrong."
Physician: "Your reports are unacceptable."
You: "Why are they unacceptable? Are they too late?"
Physician: "No. They are too difficult to interpret."
You: "You mean they are too long?"
Physician: "No. They are just hard to interpret."
You: "Is it a question of terminology?"
Physician: "You got it."
You: "If I include the old terminology in parenthesis, would that solve the problem?"
Physician: "Yes."

7. Use fogging. Fogging is agreeing in principle or agreeing with some truth in a derogatory statement. This is usually followed by disagreeing with the major thrust of the criticism. For example, "Yes, we often appear to be disorganized. However, we do know what we are doing at all times."
8. Be tentative if you doubt a statement's appropriateness: "What you say seems to make sense, but I will have to think about that."
9. Admit it if the comment seems appropriate: "You are right. I must be more careful in the future."
10. If the criticism is not valid and you do not choose to refute it, say to yourself, "That is one fallible person's opinion." If the criticism should be challenged, do it in a factual, objective, and unemotional way.
11. If the criticism is valid, thank the person (without sarcasm).
12. Admit that it bothers you: "I know there is something in what you said, and I must admit it is hard for me to accept."
13. Seek the opinion of others to confirm or disprove what has been charged.

REFERENCES

1. The 3M Meeting Management Team. *How to Run Better Business Meetings*. New York, NY: McGraw-Hill; 1987.
2. Munn HE Jr. The supervisor as a responsible listener. *Health Care Supervis*. October 1982:62-71.
3. Bandler R, Grinder J. *Frogs Into Princes: Neurolinguistic Programming*. Moah, Utah: Real People Press; 1979.
4. Covey SR. *The 7 Habits of Highly Effective People*. New York, NY: Simon & Schuster; 1990.

5. Argyle M, Dean J. Eye contact, distance, and affiliation. *Sociometry.* 1965;28:289-304.

3. Self-Esteem and Assertiveness

Two personal characteristics are sine qua non for dealing successfully with difficult people. The first, assertiveness, is needed in every encounter with problem behaviors; we will focus on this quality in this chapter. The second, stress resistance, is essential when one is faced with sustained or recurrent confrontations or vexations; we will turn to this topic in the next chapter. Before tackling the difficult issues of assertiveness and stress resistance, however, we must address the bedrock upon which these other qualities lie: self-esteem.

OPTIMISM AND SELF-IMAGE

Whether you are optimistic or pessimistic is simply a matter of how you see the world. Optimists happily claim their appellation, but not so with the pessimists. Pessimists insist that they are realists—and they really are. Optimists, on the other hand, view things through rose-colored glasses.

A person's outlook on life may have medical significance. Optimism releases endorphins (stress relievers), whereas emotions release epinephrines (stress inducers). A longitudinal investigation of Harvard students revealed that pessimists had a higher death rate and more chronic illness than optimists.[1]

Factors that impact our outlook include our self-image, how we are treated by others, our past successes and failures, and our emotional feelings. Much of our self-image is programmed during our first few years of life. We then spend the rest of our years validating that image. We copy the behavior, stereotypes, preferences, and prejudices of our parents. This parental script is modified by the expectations we develop by ourselves and by those who look up to us. It is impacted by how we talk to ourselves and from our conclusions as we compare ourselves to others, which is something we do all the time. This self-talk is largely unfavorable because we tend to match ourselves with individuals who we think are better or more fortunate than we are.

SELF-ESTEEM

"Self-esteem is a feeling of self-worth. It's being a somebody...a fundamental, universal, and pervasive human need."[2]

Self-esteem = self-efficacy + self-respect + acceptance. *Self-efficacy* is having confidence in one's ability to cope with life's challenges—a sense of control. It requires technical or professional competency, skill, and knowledge. We must feel empowered and in control of our lives and our daily work. To achieve *self-respect*, we must like and respect ourselves. In fact, we cannot like or love others until we like ourselves. Self-respect demands integrity—ethical and moral standards. The final ingredient is *acceptance* of ourselves by others, such as our colleagues, family members, teammates, or other social groups.

External Factors Affecting Self-Esteem

Self-esteem plummets in special work situations such as the first few days in a new position, during counseling or performance appraisal interviews, when criticized, when taking a test, or after losing a job. Poor or autocratic leadership that features demands for conformity, lack of performance feedback or respect, disregard for employees' opinions, denigration of accomplishments, and cronyism quickly erodes employee self-esteem.

Internal Factors Affecting Self-Esteem

Internal factors that impact our self-esteem are principally negative emotions. Being buffeted by a negative emotion is like trying to drive a car with the emergency brake on: movement is limited and great strain is put on the parts. Among the many negative emotions are the two great destroyers: fear and guilt. Our biggest fears are fear of failure, fear of rejection, and fear of being controlled by other people or things (the "victim complex"). Guilt is characterized by feelings of inferiority or inadequacy, being regarded as undeserving, or being easily manipulated by others.

Seven Strategies for Boosting Self-Esteem

1. Do not beat yourself up or let others do it to you.
Abort the negative self-talk that keeps welling up from your subconscious mind (eg, "You might have known that you were going to screw up, you jerk!"). Stop comparing yourself to other people. Be a risk taker. Regard setbacks and failures as learning experiences. Forgive yourself (and others) for everything you ever did wrong. Do it right now!

2. Use affirmations.
Affirmations are direct, one-sentence statements of a quality, characteristic, habit, or goal we wish to achieve or strong positive statements that are already true. These should not be merely idle wishes (eg, "One of these days I am going to win the lottery!"). Instead, use positive, not tentative, statements. Say "I will," not "I am going to try" or "I should." Use the present tense. Instead of "I will not cringe when Dr. Furious walks in," say, "I now feel comfortable when Dr. Furious walks in."

3. Enhance your job security.
Make yourself more marketable or indispensable. Expand and fine-tune your expertise. Upgrade your continuing education program. Train for alternative jobs.

4. Empower yourself.
Self-empowerment enables you to live your life your way—to be the authentic you. A feeling of being in control is more a perception than a reality. Avoid the "victim complex" by reflecting on all the choices and options you do have in your daily work. Accept more responsibility and earn more authority.

5. Live passionately.
Replace negative thinking patterns with positive ones. Choose one area of your life in which to be more optimistic: work, social relationships, or health.

Fill your day with enthusiasm. A popular seminar leader, Susan Dellinger,[3] recommends that we wake up with enthusiasm by clapping our hands and shouting "It's going to be a great day."

Throughout the day exhibit enthusiasm, even when you do not feel like it— "fake it 'til you make it." Add smiles to your outward display; they boost self-esteem. Your message is "You are okay, I am okay." Avoid frowns and grim facial countenances; they lower self-esteem and project pessimism. Look for the good in every situation and surround yourself with enthusiastic go-getters.

6. Take care of your body.

Exercise regularly, eat a balanced diet, and avoid alcohol, drugs, nicotine, and excess caffeine. Get involved in wellness and recreation programs.

7. Take care of your mind.

Learn how to relax or to meditate. Use supports that accept you unconditionally, such as faith, pets, hobbies, and trustworthy friends.

Practice success imagery. This is more than a visualization technique. It is mentally experiencing success, a technique that has been used extensively in sports and with people who are coping with serious medical conditions, especially cancer. The two kinds of success imagery are "results imagery" and "process imagery." When using the former, a person experiences only a final result, such as being awarded a promotion or certificate. In "process imagery" one experiences every move and sensation through the winning process, from beginning to end.

When necessary, seek professional counseling. Therapy is like getting a second opinion. It is unbiased and helps you to see the truth. A good counselor does not provide advice, but only helps you to find your own.

After you have attained a high level of self-esteem, you are ready to use this confidence to enhance your sense of assertiveness.

ASSERTIVE BEHAVIOR

Assertiveness is standing up for one's personal rights and expressing one's feelings and beliefs in direct, honest ways that do not violate the rights of others. The predominant life script for assertive people is "You are okay, I am okay."

The distinction between assertiveness and aggressiveness is sometimes blurred. The critical parameter is whether or not the rights of another person are violated. When they are, then we are talking about aggressive—not assertive—behavior.

Some assertive people speak in a forceful, dynamic manner; others, who are just as assertive, are quiet and soft-spoken. Assertive people can get things done without getting angry or emotional.[4]

Effective managers do not have to "pull rank" to get things done. They have sufficient personal power to accomplish this. Their personal power is based on knowledge, skill, experience, self-esteem, and leadership ability. Assertiveness is needed to translate this personal power into action. When you hear a manager say, "You will do as I say because I am in charge here," you are listening to a person who must rely on his authority as a manager to be seen as powerful. When a distraught mother yells at her teenage son, "I am your mother and you will do what you are told to do, young man," she does not feel in charge—and her son knows it.

The body language of assertive people features smiles and frowns, eye contact, nods and shakes of the head, firm handshakes, open and outstretched gestures, and facial expressions that express interest. Their posture is relaxed, head up, and body erect with no fidgeting or shifting weight from one foot to the other.

The verbs of assertive people include words such as, "I do not care to..."; "You are entitled to your opinion, but..."; "I have not finished my statement..."; and "Please wait your turn...." Their voice tone, which signals self-confidence, is in the midregister, volume moderate, and the rate of speed appropriate for the message.

PASSIVE BEHAVIOR

Passivity is permitting others to violate one's rights. The passive person expresses thoughts and feelings in such an apologetic manner that others can easily disregard them. The life script for these individuals is "You are okay, I am not okay."

Passive professionals, especially those with managerial responsibilities, are less respected by associates, subordinates, or superiors, and are often taken advantage of by these people.

The body language of passive people includes evasive eye contact, backing off, hunched shoulders, limpid handshakes, and covering one's mouth with one's hands. Their posture is often stiff or squirming. They tend to back up and look down.

The verbs of passive people are delivered in a timid, tremulous voice that is often weak or whining—accompanied by much sighing and throat clearing. When they speak slowly, they sound tentative. When their rate of speech is fast, they seem anxious. Verbal clues include phrases such as, "This may sound stupid, but..."; "I am sorry to have to say this..."; and "I will try."

Sometimes nonassertive behavior can result in passive-aggressive behavior, which is also referred to as hidden aggression. People usually move into this mode compulsively because of conditioning. It is a defense mechanism for survival in an environment in which the person feels powerless. It is a way to defy, retaliate, and resist offensive treatment.[5] Passive-aggressive behavior may consist of missing meetings, arriving late, taking sick days when attendance is badly needed, following instructions to the letter despite the knowledge that such action will be detrimental, and "accidentally" breaking an expensive instrument or dropping an important specimen.

AGGRESSIVE BEHAVIOR

The goal of aggression is domination and winning. The life script for this group is "I am okay, you are not okay."

Aggressive people confront by pushing forward, interrupting, glaring, and pointing fingers. They talk in loud voices, often with sarcastic or condescending overtones. Their expletives include: "I demand..."; "Listen here..."; and "You must...."

Following is an example of how these behavior types are manifested:

"Sally, this is the third morning in a row that you have been late. What is the problem?" (Assertive)
"Sally, I hate to bring this up, but you are a bit late again." (Passive)
"You are late again. You had better have a good excuse." (Aggressive)

ASSERTIVE BILL OF RIGHTS

Learn the following "Assertive Bill of Rights" before you overhaul your behavioral style:

I have the right to say what I think and feel.
I have the right to be treated with respect.
I have the right to say "no" without feeling guilty.
I have the right to ask for what I want.
I have the right to get what I pay for.
I have the right to disagree.
I have the right to be listened to and taken seriously.

If you permit others, including your boss, to violate these rights, you will not achieve assertiveness.

NINE WAYS TO ENHANCE ASSERTIVENESS

1. Feel okay about your right to act and to feel as you do.
2. Do not let others downgrade you. Eleanor Roosevelt put it well when she said, "No one can make you feel inferior without your consent." When someone puts you down, say, "Are you trying to make me feel guilty?" When they deny that, and they will, say, "Well, that is what it sounded like to me." If an associate says, "That is a dumb question," respond with, "That may be, but I still want an answer."
3. Avoid discounting or disqualifying language such as, "I may be mistaken, but..." or "I am not an expert, but...."
4. Use basic assertive statements. Simply state what you want: "Pardon me, but I would like to finish what I started to say." To a

subordinate say, "Please complete this for me," instead of, "Do you mind finishing this?"

5. Use empathic assertive statements that acknowledge the other person's opinion or feeling: "I know you do not like weekend assignments, but I must include you in the rotations."
6. Use assertive statements that express both your wants and your feelings: "When you grumble out loud about your workload, I get upset. Please stop it."
7. Once in a while use stronger language such as, "Knock that off."
8. Use assertive body language.
9. Do not turn aggressive. Be aware of the feelings and reactions of others.

SAYING NO

You must be able to say "no" and mean it. Otherwise, you will be taken advantage of not only by difficult people, but also by your friends and associates. Another activity that suffers if you can never say no is your time management: you get trapped into serving on a lot of committees, doing other people's work, and watching your open door policy being abused.

When you offer only weak refusals, you often end up saying yes. Usually it is best to say no immediately to avoid building up false hope. Say it firmly. If you have a good reason, give it. Do not apologize. Saying that you are sorry erodes your response.

Say no privately if it would embarrass the questioner. Offer alternatives: "I cannot do that, but what I can do is...." Bargain with the person by exchanging a no for a yes (eg, "Yes, I can do that for you if you will...").

The "Broken Record" technique is effective when a person will not take "no" for an answer. It is also useful in maintaining your side of an argument. For example:

> *You*: "I do not care to serve on that committee."
> *Colleague*: "You would enjoy the meetings."
> *You*: "I do not care to serve on that committee."
> *Colleague*: "You owe it to your teammates."
> *You*: "I do not care to serve on that committee."

DEALING WITH ANGER AND ANGRY PEOPLE

The most severe test of one's assertiveness is the ability to face an angry person. This will be discussed in subsequent chapters (see chapters 4, 10, and 24).

Our own anger is provoked not only by people, but also by policies, rules, rituals, procedures, deadlines, and overwork. Even equipment, such as computers, telephones, and other instruments, can provoke us, especially when they do not function. We will get into that in the next chapter.

FURTHER TRAINING

If you feel that you lack assertiveness or may be too aggressive, read at least one of the following references or suggested readings. Still better, enroll in a course or seminar on assertiveness. These are available everywhere, but you must be bold enough to sign up!

REFERENCES

1. Peterson CM, Bossio LM. *Health and Optimism*. Ann Arbor, Mich: The Free Press; 1991.
2. St. John WD. Management principles to make employees feel like somebody. *Personnel J*. 1981;60:24-26.
3. Dellinger S. *Political Savvy* [audiotape]. Boulder, Colo: CareerTrack Publishers; 1987.
4. Ash S. How to make assertiveness work for you. *Supervis Manage*. 1991;36:7.
5. Burley-Allen M. *Managing Assertively: How to Improve Your People Skills*. New York, NY: John Wiley & Sons, Inc; 1983.

SUGGESTED READINGS

Alberti RE, Emmons ML. *Your Perfect Right: A Guide to Assertive Living*. 5th ed. San Luis Obispo, Calif: Impact Publishers; 1986.

Canfield J. *Self-Esteem and Peak Performance* [audiotape]. Boulder, Colo: CareerTrack Publishers; 1987.

Fisher R, Ury W. *Getting to Yes: Negotiating Agreement Without Giving In*. New York, NY: Penguin Books; 1981.

Smith MJ. *When I Say No, I Feel Guilty*. New York, NY: Bantam Books; 1986.

Tavris C. *Anger: The Misunderstood Emotion*. New York, NY: Simon & Schuster; 1982.

Waitley D. *Denis Waitley Live on Winning* [audiotape]. Boulder, Colo: CareerTrack Publishers; 1987.

4. Stress

his chapter will provide advice on how to increase your immunity to stress and how to cope more effectively with stressful situations. You will need these supports when facing some of the difficult characters we will meet in subsequent chapters.

The signs and symptoms of excessive stress vary from person to person. Check the lists in Tables 4.1 and 4.2 to find the common medical and behavioral manifestations. The more of these symptoms you experience, the more likely you are to have a stress problem.

THE ETIOLOGY OF STRESS

Stress can be caused by many factors, chief among these are those of the human variety. However, even if we could eliminate all of our "difficult people," we still would have a stress residual caused by conflicting interests, territorial disputes, personality mismatches, and a host of nonpeople situations. See Table 4.3 for a list of common stressors.

As a boss, you can often be the source of stress for your employees. Therefore, you should avoid management strategies that inflict too much stress on your workers. Autocratic, inflexible, manipulative, and laissez-faire leadership styles all tend to foment stress. Ignoring people, nit-picking, showing favoritism, plugging in too little or too much communication, or demonstrating a lack of integrity can wreak havoc with employee self-esteem, which is the antistress breastplate.

Anxiety or depression
Chronic fatigue
Insomnia and nightmares
Headaches, backaches, premenstrual syndrome
Loss of appetite
Compulsive eating
Difficulty getting up in the morning
High blood pressure

Table 4.1   Stress or Burnout: Medical Signs and Symptoms.

Emotional outbursts
High-pitched laughter
Increased irritability
Trembling, tics, or stuttering
Decline in performance
Absenteeism
Complaints about working conditions
Resistance to change
Lack of participation in meetings
No enthusiasm
Procrastination
Talk of escaping
Increased use of alcohol or drugs

Table 4.2   Stress or Burnout: What Associates Observe.

THE FOUR TYPICAL STAGES OF COPING WITH STRESS

We usually go through four stages when we are faced with a chronic stressor or a constant barrage of multiple stressful situations:

1.   We do nothing. We anticipate that the stress will go away.
2.   We seek fast relief. We gulp down a lot of analgesics, increase our intake of alcohol, or take too many tranquilizers.
3.   We take it out on others, usually subordinates, family members, or the family pet.

| External: Work related |
| Job itself |
| Role in organization |
| Career development |
| Work relationships |
| Organizational climate |
| **External: Non–work related** |
| Family |
| Financial |
| Materialism |
| Transportation |
| **Internal: Self-induced** |
| Frustrated ambition, unattainable goals |
| Workaholic |
| Feeling of powerlessness or lack of control |
| Lack of self-esteem |
| Lack of assertiveness |
| Low stress tolerance level |
| Irrational thinking |
| The "must" imperatives |
| Stretching virtues into evils |

Table 4.3   Classification of Stressors.

4.   We work it out ourselves or we get help—or suffer burnout. See Table 4.4 for a burnout self-analysis form.

Ideally, we take measures to minimize stress or take appropriate action when we realize that stress is affecting us negatively. As in all medical conditions, prevention is best. Early diagnosis and treatment are next best.

THE IMPORTANCE OF NEGATIVE EMOTIONS

The stress produced by a constant feeling of frustration leaves people drained and exhausted at the end of the day. The negative emotions that result can shake our confidence and self-esteem; the most important ones are anger, fear, and guilt.

Ask yourself these questions:

I avoid meetings or do not participate in them as actively as before.

I spend less time with my friends or family.

I often think about escaping to a farm or some distant place.

I lack enthusiasm and feel tired all of the time.

Weekends and vacations no longer rejuvenate me.

I experience periods of depression.

I have difficulty getting up in the morning.

My family says I am more impatient or irritable.

My attendance record has gone down.

I drink more alcohol or take drugs.

I am more susceptible to illnesses.

I use medications for headaches, stomach distress, nervousness, or
   sleeplessness.

My productivity has gone down or I am making more errors.

I complain more about workloads or working conditions.

People accuse me of being more cynical or sarcastic.

I feel anger welling up inside toward my job, superiors, or coworkers.

I have difficulty making decisions and tend to procrastinate more.

I hate task or schedule changes and try to prevent them.

I eat more and am gaining weight.

Table 4.4   Burnout Self-Analysis.

Dealing With Anger

Tavris[1] made an exhaustive study of anger and found it to be a complex emotion, often representing the expression of chronic fear, anxiety, self-doubt, guilt, resentment, and frustration. Anger results when these underlying emotions get the better of us. For example: Supervisor Marie explodes when her assistant fails to attend a staff meeting. She fails to recognize that her anger is fueled by a subconscious fear that her assistant contemplates resigning.

The importance of developing insight into our anger cannot be overemphasized, since many of the difficult people we will talk about later can really ruffle our feathers. In order to best handle our anger, we need to discover what is really causing us to be angry.

Throughout our lives, we learn several inefficient ways to deal with this anger. Such questionable strategies for coping with anger include:

1. "Get it out of your system." Pop psychology invariably recommends this. Tavris[1] concluded that this regime is more likely to aggravate than to alleviate an unstable relationship. At best it provides only transient stress relief, while clumsy personal confrontations can backfire—often leading to tempestuous scenes. Another problem with "getting it out of your system" is that when the provoking agent is our boss or a customer, we are more likely to take it out on someone else—a colleague who is lower on the pecking scale or a loved one at home. Such episodes are frequently followed by intense feelings of guilt.
2. "Grin and bear it" or "turn the other cheek" are still taught at home and in church. But, when this results in emotional hurts being stored up, we begin to "gunny sack," holding in our anger inside without an appropriate outlet for our emotions. This invariably leads to eventual eruptions of intense anger—like the buildup of static electricity.
3. Mulling over an irritating incident or repeating it to anyone who will listen seldom provides the insight necessary for a healthy resolution. Such tactics are more likely to result in the development of a victim or martyr complex.

Following are intervention techniques that do work because they get at the root of the problem and enable a person to get rid of the emotional overload of the anger:

1. Analyze your anger by asking yourself these questions:
   ■ What am I really angry about?
   ■ How often does this anger manifest itself?
   ■ How intense is the anger?
   ■ What are the specific provoking stimuli: criticism, put-downs, pressure, threats, denials, or irritation?
   ■ How do I react to anger and how effective have these reactions been?
   ■ Do people only listen to me when I am angry?
   ■ Are you using anger to browbeat someone or to escape personal responsibilities—the "blaming syndrome"?
2. Discuss your anger with a trusted supporter or counselor. Attempt to ferret out background emotions.
3. Determine what you want to achieve. Is it to change or to avoid the provoking situations, to change your attitude toward the other person, or to hurt the provoker?
4. Anticipate and prepare for the next encounter. Learn to recognize and avoid your "anger triggers." Prepare what you will say or do (or not say or do) at the next confrontation.
5. Use "cooling off" thoughts or humor to deflate the anger. Abort anger by having a mental "safe harbor," which is a mental image

of a relaxing scene (seashore, farm, meadow, woods) that you are in. Visualize the surroundings, hear the sounds, feel the warm sun, and smell the flowers. All your senses are engaged. Pull into this "safe harbor" whenever you feel anger welling up. Do it right in front of the offending person. It is impossible to be angry and relaxed at the same time.

6. Walk away if you do not think you can handle the situation.
7. Learn relaxation techniques.
8. After an angry encounter write a nasty letter, put it aside, and tear it up later. If the anger persists, get your mind off of it by doing something distracting—playing sports, doing a hobby, walking in the woods, doing a crossword puzzle, playing a computer game, listening to your favorite music, or reading an inspirational or a joke book.

Dealing With Fear

We are all confronted with many fears, both real and imagined. Fear of rejection is a powerful emotion. Insecure managers may lose control of their team because they fear losing friendships. Some subordinates will eventually take advantage of these managers.

Fear of not being in control of one's life or daily responsibilities leads to chronic complaining or burnout. People who are plagued by this fear talk a lot about luck, wishes, or being at the mercy of others.

Fear of failure affects all of us to some extent. When this persists, it becomes worry—a sustained form of fear. Worry involves thinking about, talking about, and imagining exactly what it is that we do not want to happen. A striking example of this is the "Wallenda factor." Karl Wallenda, the famous tightrope aerialist, was fearless, self-confident, and poised. Then he grew timid and hesitant. He took special precautions and started double-checking his high wire. Instead of directing his energies into taking his skywalk, he concentrated on not failing. Wallenda fell to his death in San Juan in 1978.

While there are many quick-fix psychological approaches to getting rid of fears, more permanent "cures" require measures that elevate self-esteem. It is also important for us to take full responsibility for our lives and our actions. There is a direct relationship between accepting responsibility and feeling in control. When fear wells up (or is expressed by anger or frustration) say over and over to yourself: "I am responsible and I am in charge."[2]

Dealing With Guilt

Guilt is a major source of insecurity and stress. It is characterized by feelings of inadequacy, self-criticism, susceptibility to manipulation, and the urge to make others feel the same. Guilt language features "I am sorry," "It was not my fault," or "I have to."

Here are some practical coping strategies for dealing with guilt:

1. Strive for excellence, but not perfection (except for the medical instances in which zero defects are needed, such as in cross-matching of blood).
2. Do not let others make you feel guilty. Respond by saying, "Are you trying to make me feel guilty?" They will usually become embarrassed and apologize.
3. Do not take criticism personally. Concentrate on what is being criticized. Do not get defensive. Thank the critic!
4. Do not beat yourself up! Do not let minor aggravations get to you. Acknowledge the little bumps and look beyond them.
5. We often feel guilty when we goof. Regard mistakes as learning experiences. Every active person makes mistakes. The only way to avoid falls is to stay seated. Losers react by avoiding second attempts; winners come back and try again. Bounce like a golf ball, not like an egg.
6. Forgive yourself for everything you ever did that made you feel guilty. And forgive every one else for everything they might have done. This is a great sign of maturity.

STRESS SUSCEPTIBILITY AND RESISTANCE

We all have different thresholds of stress resistance. Mary goes bananas when she breaks a fingernail. Lucy, buffeted by a seemingly unending series of personal tragedies, hangs in there without batting an eye.

Certain categories of people are more susceptible to stress than others. These sensitive groups include perfectionists, workaholics, martyrs, over-achievers, nonassertive people, and anyone with low self-esteem. Low self-esteem is perhaps the single most powerful factor in stress susceptibility.

Bernstein and Rozen[3] report that managers who are resistant to stress have three characteristics in common.

1. Control. People who feel that they have control over their lives and their work are less susceptible to external forces. The high incidence of burnout among nurses has been attributed in part to what the nurses perceive as lack of control over their daily activities. They feel like puppets on strings that are pulled by patients, patients' families, medical staff, and nursing administrators.
2. Commitment. These stress-resistant folks have convinced themselves that they are in the right line of work, are associated with

the right organization, are doing the right tasks, have the right relationships, and have the right outside interests.

3. Acceptance of challenge. These individuals regard setbacks as problems to be solved rather than catastrophes. They respond to a loss in one area of their lives (eg, demotion) by taking on a challenge in another area (eg, pursuing a new career or developing an outside interest or hobby). They may seek a new employer or redouble their efforts to improve their performance at their current job.

How to Develop Stress Resistance

Stress resistance is largely a matter of high self-esteem.

> High self-esteem = a high threshold for stress
> High self-esteem = a high level of energy
> High self-esteem = a high level of optimism
> High self-esteem = a high level of enthusiasm

The importance of high self-esteem cannot be overemphasized. Self-esteem replenishes our stores of energy and slows down its rate of depletion. Self-esteem forces optimism, enhances creativity, attracts winners, builds networks, improves persuasion, and impresses bosses. Administrators regard enthusiastic people as having a positive attitude and being go-getters. One of the great things about enthusiasm is that it is infectious!

To have high self-esteem we must believe in ourselves and deliver a constant flow of positive messages to our subconscious mind to neutralize all the negative ones that reside there. For more on self-esteem, see chapter 3.

Some Great Ways to Increase Your Stress Resistance

1. Expect only success. Develop your personal positive self-fulfilling prophecy. You are what you think you are.
2. Keep a "brag sheet" or success journal of your accomplishments. Refer to it when negative thoughts get you down. These documents are also useful in preparing for performance reviews or when updating résumés.
3. Throughout the day, say positive things to yourself, such as "I like myself" or "I am a worthy person." Repeat these silent utterances hundreds of times a day for one month.
4. Surround yourself with optimistic, energetic, enthusiastic doers. Stay away from negative or complaining people. Join a "smile

and compliment" club of any type or a local Toastmaster's club. "If you hang around with turkeys, you will never soar with eagles!"

5. Maintain optimism by anticipating problems and thinking of yourself as a problem solver.
6. Look for the good in situations.
7. Refer to problems as challenges or opportunities.
8. Update your professional and managerial skills by initiating an active continuing education program.
9. Get involved in a research project or write an article for publication. Learn relaxation or meditation techniques. Take a course in assertiveness, stress management, or time management. Read or watch one of the many good books or tapes available on these subjects. Use visualization techniques. Close your eyes and picture the last great vacation you had. Use cognitive strategies such as the following: assess stressful situations realistically and take appropriate action; fight only for what is really worth fighting for; think of setbacks as learning experiences; avoid too much change too fast; attack one problem at a time; learn how to delegate and how to say "no."
10. Increase your job security by making yourself more marketable. Upgrade your résumé.
11. Expand your support network. Find at least one good listener. Get a mentor. Seek psychological supports.

Your Most Effective Emotional Supports

We all need support systems, whether they be people, situations, or activities, that help keep us grounded. Conditional supports include quality of work life, a happy marriage, friendships, and professional counseling. Unconditional supports are much more powerful. They accept you as you are, are always there for you, and stand by you through thick and thin. Spiritual faith, special people, pets, hobbies, and other special interests are the major categories of such supports.

Expand your network of supporters and seek their support when needed. Express your frustrations to a confidante. Find a good mentor.

BE A PROACTIVE MANAGER: SWITCH FROM FIRE FIGHTING TO FIRE PREVENTION

Now that you know how to deal with your own stress, apply these same strategies to your management style. Managers who manage by crisis (firefighters) have at least three features that increase their stress load. First, their plans, priorities, and management of time are flawed. Second, they delegate poorly, attempting to do everything themselves. Third, they react to problems only when the problems become critical. This all results in episodes of panic, finger-pointing, and denials.

Proactive leaders plan ahead, maintain a reserve of time and energy, delegate, and seek help when needed. They are good team players. Because they plan ahead and anticipate problems, they prevent or attack them while they are still minor or reversible. They prevent fires before they happen.

REFERENCES

1. Tavris C. *Controlling Anger* [audiotapes]. Boulder, Colo: Career-Track Publications; 1989.
2. Tracy B. *The Psychology of Achievement* [audiotapes]. Chicago, Ill: Nightingale-Conant Corp; 1987.
3. Bernstein AJ, Rozen SC. *Dinosaur Brains: Dealing With All Those Impossible People at Work*. New York, NY: John Wiley & Sons; 1989.

SUGGESTED READINGS

Axline LL. Identifying and helping the troubled executive. *Personnel.* 1987;64:40-47.

Chusmir LH, Durand DE. Stress and the working woman. *Personnel.* 1987;6:38-45.

Donnelly GF. *RN's Survival Sourcebook: Coping With Stress*. Oradell, NJ: Medical Economics Publishers; 1983.

Trager MJ, Willard S. *Transforming Stress Into Power: The Energy Director System*. Chicago, Ill: Great Performance Inc; 1988.

5. The Employee Selection Process

The best way to minimize the impact of difficult employees is to not hire them in the first place. Although candidate selection is not easy, trained interviewers can eliminate most candidates who are potential problems. If the suggestions in this chapter prevent you from hiring just one clunker, this book will have been worth its cost. How much would you give right now to get rid of that impossible subordinate you complain about every evening?

Except for candidates fresh out of school, we are not evaluating "new" employees; we are dealing with "used" ones. Like used cars, previously employed individuals have demonstrated varying degrees of reliability and performance. Some have been mistreated; others were poorly utilized by former employers. Past performance provides valuable clues to future performance.

Throughout our discussion I will refer to flags of caution that can alert you to selection hazards. If at the end of a job interview you visualize what appears to be a United Nation's flag display, be very reluctant to hire that person.

WHAT TO LOOK FOR IN RÉSUMÉS AND APPLICATIONS

Résumés are subjected to much ridicule. Typical comments are: "Résumés contain some of the world's greatest fiction" or "Résumés are nothing more than personal commercials." Nevertheless, important things are to be gleaned from these documents.

Caution flags go up when a candidate has changed jobs very frequently, the moves did not represent career progress, and the person fails to offer convincing explanations for these job hops. When moves are to jobs with lower pay, less responsibility, or requiring less competency, a large red flag is snapping in the wind. Equally significant are job changes attributed to "personal reasons" or "my boss and I had different chemistries." Job changes are okay when they represent career advances or are needed because of family matters such as an ailing parent or a spouse's job transfer.

EMPLOYMENT TESTING

Role simulations, knowledge or skill tests, and psychological questionnaires can be helpful in the interview process, and their use is increasing. Nevertheless, most employers still do not use them because of time and cost constraints, plus the fear of legal challenges on the basis of discrimination when there is a question of test validity. The best tests determine the ability of candidates to perform tasks that are listed in the position description. For example, applicants for a hematology position may be asked to interpret a blood smear; prospective instructors may be required to give a brief lecture.

How Many Interviewers for Each Interview?

The more people who interview a candidate, the greater the likelihood that one of them will detect a caution flag. Generally, the more important the job is the more interviewers are involved. However, one very skilled interviewer can usually outperform a battery of novices. A member of the personnel department usually conducts a preliminary interview. The key interviewer and the person whose opinion should carry the most weight is the person to whom the successful candidate will report—provided that that manager has been trained in interviewing skills. Ideally, the decision is by group consensus when multiple interviewers are involved. To get the maximum benefit from multiple interviews and to minimize duplication, each interviewer should prepare a different set of questions. One or more of the candidate's potential future peers may serve on the interview team. Coworkers have a vested interest in new associates and can often spot people they would like to have or not have on their team.

LEGAL CONSTRAINTS RELATED TO THE HIRING PROCESS[1]

The thrust of federal and state legislation is to ensure that hiring, retention, and promotion decisions be made only on the basis of the employee's ability to do the job. Supervisors must be aware of the legal requirement of the Equal Employment Opportunities Act and their organization's policies and practices related to it as well as the Americans With Disabilities Act.

In accordance with Title VI of the Civil Right's Act of 1964, many inquiries are interdicted by the Equal Employment Opportunities Commission (EEOC). Following is a partial list of forbidden questions:

- Age, nationality, and marital status.
- Spouse's occupation or place of employment.
- Pregnancy or plans for pregnancy.
- Child or baby-sitting arrangements. (You may ask if the person has problems getting to work, such as for callbacks.)
- Military record, except experience related to the job.
- Arrest record. (You may ask if the person has been convicted of a crime but not if he has been arrested.)
- Membership in organizations other than work-related ones.
- Religious affiliation.
- Nature, severity, or existence of physical or mental impairments.
- Worker's compensation history. (You may obtain this after hiring.)
- Questions asked only of a member of a protected group. (If you want to ask women if they can lift 50 pounds, you must ask men the same question.)

The Age Discrimination in Employment Act of 1967 as amended in 1986 prohibits employers from placing an age limit on candidates for employment except for those occupations in which age is a bona fide qualification (eg, police officer or firefighter).

The Rehabilitation Act of 1973 and the Americans With Disabilities Act of 1992 have two major aspects: those that relate to hiring and promotion practices and those that require "reasonable accommodation."

The cardinal rule is that any question asked of candidates should relate to the job in some way. You can ask whether an applicant is able to perform all job-related functions and can meet attendance requirements, but you may not ask about an applicant's current or past medical or health condition.

If an applicant reveals that he cannot perform an essential function, do not probe into his medical history. Instead, tailor the questions to identify how the disability renders the applicant unable to perform the job's essential functions and how any requested accommodations would enable the applicant to do the job.

"Reasonable accommodation" refers to measures that an employer may take to enable a person to perform essential functions. This could be physical changes such as wider doors or magnified displays. It could also involve the elimination of some nonessential or infrequently performed tasks. For example, if a job requires occasional typing, and the candidate lacks the mechanical ability to type, that activity could be assigned to other employees.

All this sounds confusing to the manager who performs only occasional employment interviews. However, one simple rule will keep you out of trouble: ask as many questions as you wish, but ask only those that will help you to determine if the person is qualified for the position being offered.

THE QUESTIONING SYSTEM

The questioning system has two equally important components: process and content.

The Questioning Process

1. Use probing sequences. These start with an introductory question followed by an in-depth series of questions related to the original one. For example:

   Introductory question: "Tell me about a work crisis you faced."
   Probing questions: "How did that situation arise?"; "Why was that allowed to happen?"; "How did you respond?"; "In retrospect, how could it have been handled better?"

2. Use hypothetical situations. For example:

   "If you suspected that one of your coworkers had a drinking problem on the job, what would you do?"

3. Early in the interview, ask some "knock-out" questions. The wrong answer to such questions eliminates a candidate before you have wasted a lot of time. For example:

   "Would you be available for weekend assignments?" (The assumption is that weekend assignments are mandatory.)

4. Do not ask loaded or leading questions. The former force a choice between two undesirable alternatives; the latter give away the answer you seek. For example:

   "Are you anti-union?" (loaded question)
   "You are willing to serve on committees, correct?" (leading question)

5. Prepare a written menu of questions and use it for each candidate to ensure completeness, uniformity, and fairness.

The Questioning Content

Questions should evaluate competency—"can do"—and determine conformity, creativity, and motivation—"will do." Conformity includes compatibility with fellow employees, manageability by you, and compliance with policies, rules, and practices. For many positions, resistance to stress is an important commodity. Evaluating knowledge, skills, and experience (competency) is relatively easy. Determining the other attributes is much more difficult.

Because questions to evaluate competence are relatively simple to formulate, I will limit the lists of recommended questions to those related to the factors of motivation, compatibility, manageability, and stress resistance.

Questions to Measure Motivation

Every department has a few clock watchers and other marginal performers who could do better if they wanted. The following questions will help to spot these goof-offs:

- What have you done that demonstrates initiative and willingness to work?
- What did you do to become more effective in your position?
- Tell me about your self-development program.
- Tell me about a time when you "went the extra mile."
- In hindsight, how could you have improved your progress?
- How do you feel about your present workload?
- Do you set goals for yourself? Tell me about your most important one.

Questions to Evaluate Compatibility

Most jobs involve teamwork. Teamwork demands communication skills, congenial relationships, cooperation, the ability to compromise, and a lot of healthy give and take. The following questions help to evaluate this important trait:

- Do you like to assume responsibility for your own work or to share the responsibility with others?
- Describe your participation in staff and committee meetings.
- With what kinds of people did you have contact and what things did you do differently with each of these different types?
- What kinds of people irritate you? How do you deal with them?
- What kinds of people do you get along with best? What kinds of people do you find difficult?
- With what other departments did you have dealings, and what difficulties did you encounter with any of these?

Questions to Evaluate Manageability

Although you are not looking for a clone of yourself, you want people who complement your strong points. It is critical to surround yourself with people who can adjust to your leadership style. You may be a "let-'em-alone" type, in which case you do not want individuals whose answers reveal that they need constant supervision and moral support. On the other hand, if you tend to be nurturing and supportive or if you like to be in complete charge, you are unlikely to have a happy relationship with a kamikaze follower. Award bonus points to a candidate who speaks highly of a previous employer, especially if that employer is known to be a tyrant. These questions should help you pick a congenial teammate:

- Describe the best boss you ever had. Describe the worst boss you ever had (watch the body language).
- In what ways did your boss contribute to your desire to leave your previous position?
- What are some of the things you and your boss disagreed about?
- What are some things your boss did that you disliked?
- Tell me about your attendance record at school and work.
- How would you describe your followership style?
- How do you feel about overtime? Call-backs? Extra-hour assignments?
- Describe your last performance review.
- Give me an example of how you handled unjust criticism.
- Did your boss delegate things to you? Tell me about a couple of those.

Questions to Evaluate Stress Resistance

Today's health care workers are under more stress than ever before. They have to deal with less job security, frequent staff shortages, more rapid changes, fear of AIDS, institutional restructuring, demands for shorter turnaround time, and the need to do more with less. In STAT labs, blood banks, special care units, and emergency rooms, the burnout rate may be very high. This burnout is observed more frequently than we care to admit. All of us have different stress thresholds, and different jobs generate different amounts of stress. If the position you are trying to fill is a stressful one, you will want to include questions such as the following:

- When was the last time you got angry at work? What caused it and how did you react?
- How would you describe a motivating work atmosphere?
- What were your biggest job frustrations?
- What was the most difficult situation you faced at work?
- What kinds of feelings did you have and how did you react to them?
- What are some of your pet peeves?
- Describe the kind of environment in which you function best.

- When you are faced with a stressful situation how do you cope with it?
- To what kinds of emotional supports do you turn?
- How do you relax or restore your energy?

CLUES TO UNTRUTHFUL CANDIDATES

If you observe any of the following qualities in a candidate, the red flag should go up immediately.

1. Their résumés and comments seem too good to be true.
2. You have difficulty believing what they said they were paid or the raises they claimed to have received.
3. They exaggerate or falsify their educational achievements (eg,"attended" becomes "graduated from").
4. Their answers to challenging questions make you dubious of what they claim or what their résumés state.
5. Their body language gives them away. They show signs of discomfort or restlessness when closely questioned, they avoid eye contact, and they may cover their mouths with a hand. You note blushing, sudden heavy perspiring, or a change in voice (pitch, volume, or rate).
6. The information you get from their references does not jibe with what they told you.

OBTAINING RELIABLE REFERENCES

Getting information from references is growing more and more difficult because human resource departments and managers want to avoid legal problems that may arise from comments they make about former employees. With a little persistence and diplomacy, however, much can be learned.

The past or present immediate supervisor of a candidate is best qualified to comment on performance. Permission must be obtained from candidates to speak to their former employers. Ask candidates to call their references to alert them regarding your intended inquiry. The references are much more likely to talk to you if this is done. If a candidate is reluctant to have you talk to former supervisors, the old caution flag is up again, unless the candidate has not yet left his current job. If that is the situation, ask for the name of a previous supervisor or request a copy of the candidate's last performance appraisal.

Following is a strategy for getting the information you seek from a potentially reluctant reference. After introducing yourself, state, "I would like to verify some information given to us by Bill Smith, who has given me permission to talk to you." This introduction, merely asking for confirmation of information, will usually elicit a positive response. Ask if this is a good time and place to talk. The person may want to go to another site for more privacy or may want to call you back later.

If the person is reluctant to say anything, or states that it is against company policy to furnish such information, say that the lack of such information may exclude the candidate from further consideration. Ask if an exception to the policy can be made in this case.

Ask for confirmation of data supplied by the candidate such as title, dates of employment, responsibilities, and salary. Then move on to the same key questions you had asked the candidate, after assuring the respondent that the information is confidential. Save the more sensitive questions for last.

Note how respondents talk about the person. If their comments are very brief, hesitant, or guarded, the caution flag is up once more.

RECENT GRADUATES APPLYING FOR THEIR FIRST PERMANENT JOB

Yate[2] puts it well when he states, "Hiring fresh college grads is like dabbling in futures—a very risky business." However, most college graduates do have employment histories of sorts. They have also not yet learned any bad habits and are often eager to prove themselves at work. Many have had part-time or summer jobs. A few were full-time employees before attending college or had interrupted their education to work for a time. Inquiries into these employment experiences should be made, and the same panels of questions used. The following questions assume greater importance when the employment history is skimpy:

- Which of your school years (or subjects) was the most difficult? Why?
- With which teachers did you have problems? Why?
- What are some of the problems you faced at school or at home? If you had it to do all over, what would you do differently?
- What are the advantages and disadvantages of your chosen field?
- What kind of work interests you the most?
- Tell me about any jobs you have had, paid or voluntary.
- What have you done that shows initiative and willingness to work?
- What future educational endeavors do you have in mind?
- What job in our organization would you like best? Why?

IMPORTANCE OF INTUITION IN THE SELECTION PROCESS

Many managers are reluctant to admit that intuition plays a role in their selection process. However, it is now the "in" thing to confess that you are influenced by those little messages that pop up from your subconscious mind. And not only is intuition a popular topic but it is also a valuable tool. Numerous studies have demonstrated the value of intuition. The most expert decision makers make full use of both their rational and their innovative capabilities. Most, if not all, of those "aha" thoughts that break through—often when we least expect them—are not flashes from outer space but are based on experiential information stored deep in the catacombs of our subconscious minds.

This does not mean that we should act on all of these "aha's." What they do is to alert us to the need to focus our rational thought process on a particular aspect. For example, suppose you are interviewing a candidate who has outstanding credentials and is handling his end of the interview flawlessly—asking all the right questions, giving all the right answers, and showing keen interest in the job—but you are experiencing a series of discomforting vibes. Try to ferret out the reason for these feelings. Maybe you feel intimidated or threatened; maybe you are turned off by his long hair or informal attire—observations that should not disqualify the person for most jobs. However, maybe the person seems a little too glib. So, you put in a few extra challenging questions and follow up with more probing queries.

On rare occasions you cannot find anything wrong, but you still have a strong feeling that you would not hit it off with this person. This is a good time to get input from other observers. Schedule a couple more interviews for that purpose.

TAKE FULL ADVANTAGE OF THE PROBATIONARY PERIOD

An almost universal failing of managers is to give marginal performers the benefit of the doubt at the end of their probationary period—only to regret it later. The excuse that is usually given is that the person just needs more experience or that you will smooth out his rough edges later.

There are at least two effective ways to avoid this pitfall. The first is to pay more attention to the performance of new hires, provide frequent feedback to them, and evaluate their ability and willingness to shape up. All too often, the time slips by and one dreary morning your human resources department calls for your evaluation of that new person.

The other tactic is simply to request an extension of the probationary period, citing either marginal performance to date or that the complexity of the job demands a longer period of observation. Most human resource departments will permit this. During the extended observation period, make every effort to determine the new hire's "can do" and "will do" capabilities.

REFERENCES

1. Umiker W. *Management Skills for the New Health Care Supervisor.* 2nd ed. Gaithersburg, Md: Aspen Publishers; 1993.
2. Yate M. *Hiring the Best: How to Staff Your Department Right the First Time.* 3rd ed. Holbrook, Mass: Bob Adams Inc; 1990.

SUGGESTED READINGS

Arthur D. *Recruiting, Interviewing, Selecting & Orienting New Employees.* New York, NY: AMACOM; 1986.

Fear R. *The Evaluation Interview.* 3rd ed. New York, NY: McGraw-Hill; 1984.

Feuer D, Lee C. The Kaizen connection: how companies pick tomorrow's winners. *Training.* 1988;25:23-35.

Fritz NR. Culture clash. *Personnel.* 1988;65:6-8.

Half R. *Half on Hiring.* New York, NY: Crown Publishing; 1985.

Parks DG. Employment references: defamation law in the clinical laboratory. *Clin Lab Manage Rev.* 1993;7:103-110.

Smart B. *The Smart Interviewer.* New York, NY: John Wiley & Sons; 1989.

Stanton ES. Telephone reference checks. *Personnel J.* 1988;67:123-130.

Swan WS. *How to Pick the Right People.* New York, NY: John Wiley & Sons; 1989.

6. Better Orientation and Training of New Employees

If you fill job vacancies with carefully selected candidates you can eliminate many potential problems. The suggestions in the last chapter will help you sort out the bad risks. Unfortunately, in some instances there is a dearth of good candidates, and we must pick with reluctance and trepidation. This state of affairs increases the importance of preparing new employees for their new responsibilities. An effective orientation and training program is a powerful proactive supervisory tool for increasing the likelihood of satisfactory performance and avoiding the possibility of dysfunctional behavior. In this chapter, we will discuss the particulars involved in turning new hires into effective colleagues.

THE ORIENTATION PROGRAM

New hires are eager, willing, and susceptible to indoctrination. Werther[1] expresses this as follows: "At no other time is there a better opportunity to open lines of communication with new hires. They are free from the distortions of peer groups; they have not yet formed strong opinions about the job, company, or boss; and they are so eager to please."

You only get one chance to take advantage of this opportunity. A botched orientation program, weak training, or exposure to senior employees who have a poor work ethic can start a new employee down a spiraling path to poor performance, negative attitude, and job dissatisfaction.

When Does An Orientation Program Start?

A program actually shifts into first gear when people are interviewed for jobs. In most instances, their initial impressions were favorable, since they have accepted your offer.

In progressive organizations, contacts are also made between the date of acceptance and the date of arrival. These contacts may be as simple as a congratulatory phone call. Invitations to lunch or to some other type of get-acquainted meeting are more impressive, demonstrate caring, and help to minimize the first-day-on-the-job jitters. As Yate[2] states, "For the new hire, the first week is often marked not so much by enjoyment and camaraderie as by something approaching terror."

Your orientation program is more likely to succeed if you:

- Tell the new employees exactly what they are to do.
- Tell them how well and how quickly these things must be done.
- Show them how to do the things with which they need help.
- Let them know how they are doing.
- Reward them for good performance—heavy on praise, light on criticism.
- Treat them as associates, not subordinates.

Yate[2] recognizes, "We made a bigger fuss over a new machine than we did over the person we hired to operate it. And our employees, who were not stupid, began to notice."

The Mission of a Good Orientation Program

The following six goals are crucial to ensuring the success of an orientation program:

1. To create a favorable impression of the organization, your department, and the managers, especially you.
2. To orient new employees to the big picture—how their group fits into the organization—and to the local picture—the part they play.
3. To establish rapport through collegial communication with emphasis on teamwork, creativity, and participation in planning, decision making, and problem solving.
4. To build confidence and self-esteem by providing initial experiences that result in early successes.
5. To inculcate the values of honesty, pride, multidirectional communication, work ethic, and customer service.
6. To satisfy the new employee's need for affiliation (friendship), achievement (job satisfaction), and control (feeling empowered).

Who is Responsible for the Orientation Program?

Most of us have no control over our organization's general ori▨ program, which is usually provided by the human resources ▨▨part-ment. However, the person to whom the new employee reports has the responsibility for orienting that person within the work unit. This should be a top priority, not to be taken lightly, despite the time con-straints due to the work group having been understaffed while the posi-tion was vacant.

Experienced and well-motivated senior employees who like to instruct—and are given enough time—can help with orientation. However, they must be patient, willing to listen to the new person's past experience, and know how to tailor instructions to individual needs.

Preparations for the New Arrival

1. Send a letter of welcome to indoctrinees. Include verification of date, time, and place of reporting, the first day's agenda, and any special instructions or suggestions, such as what they should bring or wear. Check with your human resources department for any documents that may be required.
2. Prepare an orientation packet that includes the following: departmental mission statement, goals, and organization chart; copies of the position description, work standards, and perfor-mance appraisal forms; handbook of policies and procedures; schedules of orientation and training; check-off lists of tasks that must be learned; names, titles, and locations of trainers; and key telephone numbers or condensed telephone directory. (Note: Many organizations have eliminated handbooks either because of fear of litigation or because they have found that supervisors do a better job of orientation when it must be done in person. Thick manuals and handbooks are intimidating and poor substitutes for personal discourse.[2])
3. Arrange your schedule so you can spend most of the first day with the orientee.
4. Alert others who are involved in the training program about the new employee's arrival.

The First Day

The first day is not the time to impress a new person with your importance by looking busy. Greet your new hires as you would welcome visiting friends.

If the following questions were not answered during preemployment interviews, ask them now. The responses you get will help you in making assignments and in avoiding future problems:

- Do you like taking full responsibility for your work or do you prefer group work?
- What do you think of workstation rotation? Cross-training?
- Do you like administrative responsibilities (teaching, committee work, research, etc)?
- How do you feel about overtime and weekend work?
- What do you hope to accomplish during your first year on the job?

The Attitude and Planning Talk[3]

Have a well-prepared "attitude and planning" speech, and deliver it with enthusiasm. Tell the orientees that they were selected not only because they have the necessary expertise, but also because they had shown that they were customer-focused. This is a good time to point out that your customers include patients, clinicians, visitors and parents of patients, any departments or committees served by your section, third-party payers, students and trainees, and any others. Add that you are aware that the newcomers have demonstrated in their past posts that they were hardworking, innovative, and flexible—all traits that you hope will be continued. Review the agenda of the orientation program and issue each person an indoctrination packet and locker.

The "Nuts and Bolts" Talk[3]

On the second day, ask the orientee how the first day went. Then review her position description and work standards. To emphasize the importance of these documents, refer to them as contracts that must be honored. Discuss "survival information" like work hours, overtime, compensatory time, vacation and sick leave policies, and completion of personnel data. When do they get paid and where? When and where do they take breaks and have lunch? To whom do they report? Who can provide different kinds of advice? Issue them "road maps" to help them find their way around the building and compound. Emphasize any important personnel policies of which they should be aware, such as those involving smoking in the workplace, sexual harassment, or personal safety requirements.

Now is also an excellent time to describe your likes and dislikes. It is better to alert people before they do the things that annoy you or that must be corrected. Here are some appropriate topics:

- How do you, the supervisor, want to be addressed? Do you want to be called by your first name or more formally?
- Explain your open door policy. May they walk into your office at any time? When is your door open? Only at certain times?
- Emphasize that you welcome suggestions, comments, and even criticism. Say, "In this department, we do not kill the messengers of bad tidings."
- Mention specific things that bother you (eg, tardiness, absenteeism, untidy personal appearance, and verbal expressions such as, "That is not in my position description" or "I only work here").
- Explain your policies regarding tidy desks, smoking, or having food at work stations.
- Discuss your quality assurance program and how it affects the new hire.
- Encourage the orientee to find a mentor. Mentors are experienced people who are willing to share their wisdom and/or their political clout with protégés. They become unofficial advisors, supporters, and confidantes.

"Show and Tell" Time

Do not try to cover everything during a single tour of the premises; this is too confusing for new people. Throughout the orientation program you must guard against information overload. Point out the physical facilities and major pieces of equipment. During this tour, do not stop to introduce all the employees. Do this later. In large institutions or departments, this may be done over several days during the first week.

Show new employees where things are filed or stored. Point out where schedules are posted. Direct attention to the communication systems and demonstrate their use (eg, telephones, intercom, copiers, fax machines, computers). Stress the importance of proper telephone etiquette. Illustrate how the different work shifts communicate with each other. Point out the location and proper use of safety equipment and review your safety policies. New people are concerned about the risks of contracting infectious diseases, especially viral hepatitis and AIDS. Discuss these even when no concerns have been voiced. Describe the preventive measures that must be followed.

Meeting Coworkers

I recommend against a lot of introductions at work stations. Employees do not like to be interrupted while they are concentrating on their work, and this may be perceived by the new person as unfriendliness. Also, orientees are confused by the plethora of faces, names, and titles when presented in rapid succession. Make the introductions during breaks, when workers are relaxed and more inclined to be amiable. Also, present newcomers at a staff meeting. Encourage them to talk about their educational background, work experience, and recreational activities. The new employee should also meet individually with each senior member of the department. Introduce the newcomer to key people in other departments that must coordinate with yours. Refer to such departments as important internal customers.

Recent graduates require a more detailed agenda. They are used to a highly structured program designed by their faculty, with regularly scheduled examinations. They must be made aware of the difference between such examinations and performance appraisals. Encourage them to design their personal continuing education programs, including the formulation of goals, objectives, and plans.

THE TRAINING PROGRAM

Training is More Than Developing Skills

Training is aimed not only at building skills but also at instilling healthy mental attitudes and values. We want to do more than meet our customers' expectations; we want to exceed them. When a physician leaves the laboratory with the information she sought, she should also come away with the feeling that everyone bent over backwards to please her. Teaching a clerk how to answer the telephone is skills improvement; teaching that person how to please callers is attitude development. Positive attitude should "piggy-back" on skills improvement. The best kind of attitudinal training is derived from team leaders who model the desired behavior—those who "walk the talk."

Teaching vs Learning

Teaching is not the same as learning. An animal trainer once claimed that he had taught his dog how to whistle. When he was challenged, he replied that he had indeed taught the dog how to whistle, but the dog had not learned how to do it. For training to become learning, instructors must get feedback from trainees indicating that learning has occurred.

Preparations for Training

First, make a list of all the skills necessary to do the work. Then find out which of these skills the employee already has. Do not accept what you read in résumés or heard during preemployment interviews. Ask technical or professional questions or watch the employee perform. Separate learning needs into those that can be picked up while at the worksite and those that must be taught formally. Develop a timetable for achieving educational goals.

Control of the Training Process

The control aspect of training is the most sensitive portion. While you must supervise closely enough to prevent major mistakes, you must tolerate a few minor mishaps. A common complaint of trainees is that the only feedback they get is negative, despite the fact that even the most inept new hire does most things right. Reflect on what comments you issued at your last one-on-one training session. How many were positive and how many negative? Some behavioral authorities claim that a ratio of 4 positives to 1 negative must be maintained to preserve self-esteem and motivation.

Try substituting the "enhancing value" technique for the usual form of criticism. Instead of jumping in with "No, no, that is not the way," or "Here, let me show you how to do that," start out with a positive observation to show that you are acting as a supporter rather than a critic. For example:

"Alice, I like the enthusiasm you demonstrated in that phone conversation. The caller must have been impressed; and (avoid a "but" at this point because it wipes out what preceded it), Alice, it would sound more professional if you ended with 'thank you for calling' instead of 'bye, bye.' "

Instructors must encourage creativity rather than strict conformity. Employees start down the road to attitude problems when they hear, "Forget what you learned at your previous job, you are not working there now," "Do it our way and you will get along fine," or "That is a stupid remark." These become double whammies when said in condescending or sarcastic tones. Instead, build on the people's experience and encourage them to use that experience to solve problems.

Tips for Better Training

1. Plan a highly structured process. The trainee should know what is to be learned each day, who will do the instructing, and what they should study before the next day's session. They should also know what to do between teaching sessions (eg, study handbook and procedure manuals or perform duties they have already mastered).
2. Help them to develop a success habit by working on easier skills first.

3. Talk softly—this denotes friendliness. Sit next to, not across from, the person.
4. Give examples. Use analogies. Relate hero and horror stories. Hero stories are episodes that the department is proud of, when one or more employees did something that everyone was proud of, such as being the first laboratory to offer a special service that was made possible only by the special effort of the "hero." Horror stories are when something bad happened because of carelessness or ignorance, such as when a patient dies as the result of a botched blood transfusion.
5. Correct errors before they become habits but do not nitpick.
6. Address errors, not traits or personalities. Regard mistakes as learning experiences. Relate some of your own past mistakes.
7. Be patient. Do not overwhelm the trainee. Expect to have to repeat things. Avoid an exasperated facial expression when you explain things the second or third time.
8. Treat trainees as knowledgeable adults.
9. Do not say "Any questions?" or "Do you understand?" to determine if learning has occurred. Instead, ask specific questions, give quizzes, or ask the trainees to paraphrase what you told them.
10. Verbalize your role and offer of help (eg, "I will always be available to help you," or "Do not hesitate to ask me questions at any time").

Feedback from Orientees

Have the trainees fill out a critique of the orientation program. Ask what was most valuable, how they are going to use the information they received, how you can help more, and what educational topics would be of interest to them in the future.[2]

"Graduation"

A thorough orientation and training program requires much mental effort and psychological stress on the part of trainees. Therefore, the last day of the program should be a special one for them. Three events are appropriate to celebrate this graduation:

1. Their immediate supervisor reviews with them check-off lists and critiques to ensure that everything has been covered. Congratulations are expressed enthusiastically.
2. The department chief meets with them and also congratulates them. She should know enough about their performance to date

to be able to comment on any special attributes that each trainee demonstrated during the indoctrination process. The chief reminds the trainees that henceforth they are responsible for their own continuing education program, but that staff members are always ready to assist them in their efforts.

3. A celebration of sorts is held in their honor. While a special dinner is nice, a much simpler event, such as coffee and doughnuts, will suffice. This may be combined with a routine staff meeting.

REFERENCES

1. Werther WB. *Dear Boss*. New York, NY: Meadowbrook Press; 1989.
2. Yate M. *Keeping the Best*. Holbrook, Mass: Bob Adams Inc; 1991.
3. Umiker W. *Management Skills for the New Health Care Supervisor*. Gaithersburg, Md: Aspen Publishers; 1988.

7. Coaching to Prevent Personnel Problems

Good coaching represents a proactive approach to dealing with employee problems. It reduces the number of difficult subordinates and rallies the support of team members when difficult members must be confronted. Good coaches are perceived by their employees as people who help them get their work done and who fight to defend or protect them. The resulting environment is one that prevents the development of negative attitudes and minimizes the degree of their undesired behavior. Bad coaches, on the other hand, create morale problems that lead to dysfunctional behavior, high rate of personnel turnover, and the welcoming of union activities by disgruntled employees. An effective coach functions as a trainer, facilitator, counselor, consultant, delegator, supporter, problem solver, coordinator, peacemaker, evaluator, enforcer, and disciplinarian. The coach is also the morale officer, responsible for developing an environment that motivates. A coach ensures that an unwritten "Employee Bill of Rights" is respected. Such a bill should include the following rights:

- Fair and equal treatment.
- Basic dignity and respect.
- Preservation and enhancement of self-esteem.
- Performance feedback.
- Input of employees into decisions that relate to their work.
- Collaboration of employees in setting their work goals.
- Opportunity to develop skills to meet new challenges.
- Bidirectional vertical/horizontal communication.

Coaching is more difficult now because contemporary employees are different.[1] Today's skilled employees have a choice of employers. They are less concerned about job security and less tolerant of authoritarian leadership. Most of them place family and leisure above work. They often display more loyalty to their profession than to their employer. They expect meaningful work that impacts their personal goals, not just the goals of their department. They expect more than increased salary and benefits as rewards. They want more input into decision making and departmental planning.

The bottom line is that today's workers require supervisors who are not only professionally or technically competent, but who also have strong leadership skills. They want to be led, not managed!

PRINCIPLES OF PRACTICAL MOTIVATION

1. Accept the employees. You cannot change or motivate people. Only people can motivate themselves. You can, however, change your perception of them. You can modify their behavior. You can improve morale and motivation by changing work environments and your leadership style. You can encourage employees to channel their motivation in the direction of the organization's goals.

2. Treat employees as winners. Never label anyone a loser; people are only winners and potential winners. The theory of the self-fulfilling prophecy has been proven over and over. If you convince yourself and the other person that he is a winner, then that person will perform as a winner. Consciously and subconsciously we deliver messages that boost the self-esteem and confidence of these individuals, and this is reflected in their behavior.

3. Show employees what to do, how to do it, and why it should be done. Let them know how well they are performing.

4. Praise generously and criticize sparingly. A great source of employee dissatisfaction is the lack of appreciation or recognition. Motivation requires many positive strokes to neutralize a negative one.

5. Never ignore. Even negative strokes (eg, reprimands) are more acceptable than no strokes at all.

6. Decrease dissatisfaction through empowerment. Empowerment enables people to develop personally and professionally so that their contributions in the workplace are maximized.[2] Empowerment is achieved when you:

   ■ Value innovation and creativity over conformity.
   ■ Build self-confidence by providing challenging, achievable responsibilities.
   ■ Enhance self-esteem by making people feel important.

- Ask your employees for their opinions and involve them in important decision making.
- Provide recognition for employees' efforts.

7. Reward the behavior and results that you want. Two old adages apply: "What gets rewarded gets done" or "You get what you stroke." Rewarding desired behavior helps prevent the development of troublesome relationships and reinforces positive performance.

WHAT YOU REWARD IS WHAT YOU GET

External rewards are those that someone grants. These include salary increases, bonuses, promotions, special perquisites such as an office or desk, opportunities to increase personal development, closer work ties with the boss, praise, and recognition. Internal rewards are those that people give to themselves. They include a sense of self-fulfillment, importance, or growth, increased self-esteem, a feeling of achievement, and congenial relationships with coworkers. Supervisors can help employees recognize such rewards through skillful coaching and mentoring. Positive feedback is essential.

Many supervisors unconsciously reward undesired behavior and penalize good behavior. For example, Supervisor Sue has difficulty getting Joe to do anything out of the ordinary. Joe's response to new assignments is, "That is not in my position description" or "That is your job, not mine." Sue rewards Joe and penalizes her best employee, Steve, by dumping all the busy work on Steve. Other examples of disincentives are given in Table 7.1.

---

1. John does a great job with a difficult task. Instead of a reward, such as a prized assignment, he gets another tough assignment that he dislikes.
2. Sue suggests a better way to maintain an inventory. Contrary to her wishes, she is put in charge of the stockroom.
3. Steve makes a suggestion at a staff meeting. His boss pokes fun of it.
4. Gloria admits making a mistake when she could have concealed it. She gets chewed out.
5. Bill reports a safety hazard. His boss yells, "Why do you always bring me bad news?"

Table 7.1   Examples of Punishing Good Performance.

Some employees are masters at getting attention through undesirable behavior; every school classroom has at least one of these. For example, Sue could not understand why Lucy often showed up late for work. Then one day she overheard Lucy say to a friend that the only time Lucy gets any recognition from Sue is when she is chewed out for coming in late.

ESSENTIALS OF PRAISING AND REPRIMANDING

Praising and reprimanding are such vital parts of positive feedback that they merit more detailed description.

What You Should Praise

1. Work that is above and beyond the call of duty: worked extra long hours or returned to work after hours; substituted for a sick coworker; got you out of a sticky situation; solved a difficult problem.
2. Work or behavior that is not outstanding but is always dependable: excellent attendance record; does not cause problems; is flexible and cooperative; accepts extra or unpleasant assignments.
3. Subpar work that improves (do not wait for it to reach the level of your expectations).
4. An innovative idea that is suggested.
5. A customer complaint that is passed on to you. Your impulse will be to make a face and mumble something about "another problem" or "is that all you ever bring to me?" Instead, you should thank the bearer of bad news and ask him what he thinks should be done.
6. An employee's inner qualities as well as what they accomplish: instead of saying, "Alice, you did a good job with this report," Sue says "Alice, I admire your talent for preparing difficult reports; this one is great."

When Not to Praise

1. When praise is not deserved.
2. When praise is insincere or manipulative.
3. When it would embarrass you, the recipient, or others.

How to Praise

1. Do it as soon as possible after the act. Otherwise, you may forget it or the recipient thinks that it cannot be very important.

2. Be specific so the person knows exactly what is being praised, finds it more believable, and appreciates the fact that you know what is going on.
3. Say how you feel about what was done or why it was important (eg, "When you come up with such good solutions for problems, I feel confident that you can handle things very well when I am not around").
4. Shake hands and repeat your "thank you."

Negative Feedback vs Hostile Criticism

Negative feedback (constructive criticism) is directed at behavior or work results, is helpful because it includes specific advice on how the person can do better, does not belittle, and implies confidence in the person. Hostile criticism attacks the person, contains no helpful advice, belittles, and shows lack of confidence in the person.

How to Reprimand

As in the case of praises, reprimands should: (1) follow the undesired behavior or results as soon as possible; (2) be specific; and (3) include statements of how you feel about it. Blanchard and Johnson[3] follow these three steps with an affirmation of how much you value the person and an expression of your confidence in his future performance. Following the reprimand, the person should be treated as he is on any other day. This helps the individual to realize that it was what he did (or did not do) that displeased you, and not the person himself.

How to React to Mistakes

Managers should encourage innovation and risk taking even though it means that more mistakes may occur. Only immobile people do not make mistakes. If you read the biographies of all our great inventors, political leaders, and CEOs, you find numerous confessions of not only minor but also major bad decisions, often costing millions of dollars. Not to make mistakes means never to make decisions.

If you punish mistakes, people will either avoid future risks or will conceal their blunders. Show respect for the person by reassuring him, avoiding negative messages or body language, and demonstrating a caring attitude. Look for solutions and options—not for blame. Regard mistakes as learning experiences both for you and the employees who make them.

Five Tips for Reacting to Mistakes
1. Share one of your own previous blunders.
2. Do not cross-examine. Ask "What happened?" or "How did it happen?" not "Why did it happen?" Ask what was done to fix it: "Where do we go from here?" or "How can we prevent this in the future?"
3. Select your words carefully. Use "I" not "you" language. This focuses on the behavior instead of on the person. Say, "I get annoyed when people make the same mistake over and over," not "You are too careless." Do not get caught with an unproved diagnosis: "Your trouble is that you are always in a hurry."
4. Address solutions rather than blame. Instead of, "You sure made a mess of this project," say "How do you suggest that we get out of this mess?"
5. Do not compare the person who made the mistake with others: "Why can't you be more like Mary?"

MANAGING-BY-WANDERING-AROUND[4]

Managing-by-wandering-around (MBWA) is keeping in close touch with the people who report to you—those whom you serve and those who serve you. MBWA is better than an open door policy because you leave your office and go out where the action is. You camp out with your troops.

MBWA is not just walking by with a big smile and saying hello. It is stopping for a few minutes and talking to people about work, and sometimes about their family and outside interests.

MBWA is not interrupting, holding a white glove inspection, or catching people doing something wrong. It is catching people doing something right and praising them for it.

MBWA is providing support—asking how you can help.

MBWA is asking for suggestions or complaints and jotting them down in a little book—and then doing something about them.

REFERENCES

1. Roseman E. Motivating the contemporary employee. *MLO*. 1989;21:61-65.
2. Peiffer IL, Dunlap JB. Increasing productivity through empowerment. *Supervis Manage*. 1990;35:11-12.
3. Blanchard K, Johnson S. *The One-Minute Manager*. New York, NY: Berkley Books; 1981.
4. Peters T, Austin N. *A Passion for Excellence*. New York, NY: Random House; 1985.

8. Counseling Difficult Employees

There are two kinds of counseling: career counseling when the counselor serves as an advisor or mentor and remedial counseling when a supervisor deals with employee performance that has strayed from established norms. The goal of remedial counseling is to correct deviant performance while preserving the self-esteem of the individual. The confrontation provides the person being counseled with an opportunity to look at her behavior and to decide whether or not to change that behavior. The goal should never be to release anger or frustration or to punish the employee.[1] Unsuccessful counseling usually culminates in disciplinary measures or separation.

THE THREE MAJOR KINDS OF PROBLEMS

1. Underperformance; unsatisfactory productivity or work quality.
2. Bad work habits or violation of policies or rules.
3. Inability to get along with others.

Note: When an employee is terminated because of a reduction in force or because of underperformance, that employee is entitled to unemployment compensation in most states; however, when an employee is fired because of inappropriate behavior, that employee is not entitled to this compensation.

WHERE MANAGERS GO WRONG

- They do not take action.
- They are not aware of the problem.
- They ignore the problem.
- They postpone action until the next performance review. (Employees should not have to wait until performance appraisal time to learn that they are not performing up to expectations.)
- They assume that the problem is one of poor attitude.
- They fail to monitor postmeeting behavior.
- They fail to escalate from counseling to disciplining when no improvement occurs or relapses continue.

WHY EMPLOYEES VIOLATE RULES[1]

- They never learned the rules or they forgot them.
- They see the rules as meaningless or too restrictive.
- They note that the rules are rarely or unevenly enforced.
- They are influenced by others.
- They found that the rewards of misbehavior are higher than the risks or the penalties.
- They are misfits or malcontents.

WHEN NOT TO COUNSEL

- When the problem is outside of the workplace (eg, you are told that an employee is using illegal drugs after work hours and off the premises).
- When you lack the authority to act.
- When policy restricts you from acting.
- When the behavior has no demonstrable ill effects.
- When it is not your responsibility.
- When you or the other person is emotionally upset.

PREPARING FOR THE INTERVIEW

A confrontation enables the employee to look at her behavior and decide whether or not to change.

1. Be certain that you know exactly what you want to accomplish. Ask yourself, "How does this behavior affect productivity, service quality, costs, other people, or me?"; "What if everyone did that?"

2. Be certain of the content and context of any policy or rule that has been violated. Study the document yourself, word for word.
3. Gather supporting facts. Review the employee's position description and last performance review. Check her personnel file for previous notations relating to the same problem. Get objective observations from others. Look for patterns. In the case of absenteeism, for instance, individuals may be avoiding days on which they are scheduled to do projects that they detest.
4. Explore the perceived benefit/risk ratio of the behavior from the employee's viewpoint. Are there any positive or negative reinforcers? For example, is the employee ignored when she behaves well but does she get a lot of attention when acting out?
5. If you are inexperienced in these matters, consult with a member of the human resources department. If the problem is a serious one, discuss it with your boss.
6. Construct a clear statement of your expectations for the future, and pick a realistic deadline for improvement.
7. Do not procrastinate. Think of the damage that is taking place while you are hesitating.
8. Schedule the meeting early in the morning so you have the rest of the day to show the person by your interactions that you do not bear a grudge toward her, only toward the behavior. Smile and chat just as you would if there had not been a problem discussed.
9. Pick a location where there will be no interruptions. Find an out-of-the-way conference room that you can reserve. Your office may not be a good choice.
10. Mentally rehearse these aspects of the upcoming meeting: your exact opening remarks; statements you will use to boost the employee's self-esteem; the solution you hope to find; and how you will respond to rebuttals, defensiveness, anger, tears, or threats.

THE COUNSELING INTERVIEW

The theme of the initial remedial session should be one of helpfulness. When a series of counseling sessions for the same problem follows, friendly support gives way to a sterner, more businesslike atmosphere with decreasing patience and empathy.

The Eight Steps in a Constructive Interview

1. Greet the person with a smile. Get right to the point but do not start with an intimidating statement. Remember that the first

objective is to find out if she is aware of the deviant behavior, especially if a policy or rule is being violated. Therefore, be tentative. This is even more important if there is some question of the validity of the alleged behavior. Here are two bland introductory remarks: "There is something bothering me, Joyce. I would like to discuss it with you"; "Joyce, I have a problem and I need your help."

2. Assume that the person wants to do a good job—and say so. Describe the situation in specific, nonjudgmental terms. Do not hesitate to express your feelings. Never apologize for calling the person in. You weaken your position when you start with, "I hate to bring this up, but...."

3. Explain how the behavior affects your department, other people, or you. Describing the impact of the person's behavior on you is effective because most of your employees do not want to be disliked by you or to create problems. Empathize. Admit that her job is not an easy one. Focus on the behavior rather than on the person. Use "I" language and follow with a description of the behavior. For example: "Lois, I have noticed an increasing pattern of tardiness. These late arrivals have varied from 10 to 30 minutes, two or three times a week for the past month." This statement is much better than, "Lois, you have got to do something about your tardiness."
Do not use absolute words such as "always" or "never." These words are almost always inaccurate and invite contradiction (eg, "You are never on time," is countered with, "I am usually on time"). Avoid quotations from policy manuals unless the employee challenges the authenticity of your charge. Taking refuge in a handbook makes you appear weak. For the same reason, do not say, "Management expects..."; do say "I expect...." Avoid sarcasm, kidding, or other put-downs. These elicit resentment and serve no useful purpose. Insert praise when possible.

4. Give the employee time to respond. Let her stay at it until she runs out of gas. Do not interrupt, even if she utters untruths or makes counter charges. Do not become defensive or lose your cool. Use your best listening skills. Prove that you understood what was said by paraphrasing and summarizing. Jot down the key points she makes. You may need to refer to these later.

5. Get her to admit that there is a problem and that she is a part of it. Ask her what she thinks the effects of this continued behavior will be. This forces her to focus on the possible consequences. Summarize the causes or excuses she gives: "You are saying that the parking situation is bad. I can appreciate that. However..."; "You have brought up some interesting factors. Let's look at a couple of them."

6. State that the problem must be solved, that it is up to her to solve it, and that you are there to help. If you cannot accept her first offering, keep asking for alternatives until she comes up with one that you can live with. Avoid directive phrases such as "If I were you…" or "Here is what you should do." Urge her to come up with as many solutions as she can. Discuss the pros and cons of each. If discussion stalls, ask some leading questions to guide her to additional alternatives. Do not impose your solutions unless absolutely necessary. Compliment her for coming up with solutions.

7. Summarize what is agreed upon. State your expectations clearly and empathetically. Insist on her commitment and include a deadline for the solution to take effect. Offer to help, if that is appropriate. For example, "Janet, we have agreed that it is up to you to be more courteous on the phone. If I note less than acceptable phone manners on your part, I will remind you as soon as you hang up, okay?"

8. End on a positive note with an affirmation. Thank the employee for cooperating and express confidence in her ability to solve the problem. It is often a good idea to set up a follow-up date.

Why You Should Not Offer Solutions

- Quick solutions by you make the employee feel stupid.
- When your solution does not work (and it usually will not), it will make you look stupid.
- The employee may feel that she had better solutions or she may know that your solution will not work, but she still takes it.
- Authorship means ownership. The employee will try harder when it is her solution.
- The employee does not learn how to solve her problems without help.

Roadblocks to Successful Counseling

Keep in mind that any unpleasant behavior on the part of the employee during the interview represents behavior that the individual has found effective in the past.

1. *The Employee Balks at Any Discussion*
   - She says she does not want to discuss the matter right now.
   - She denies everything you say.
   - She does not listen or keeps interrupting.

- She talks louder and faster.
- She clams up and will not say anything.
- She storms out of your office.

2. *The Employee Tries to Minimize the Problem*
- She retorts sarcastically, "Big deal" or "Okay, I have not been the employee-of-the-month; I will try to do better if that will make you happy." Never accept this. Say that you are glad that she recognizes that there is a problem and that she must realize that it is an important problem—one that you insist will be overcome.
- She challenges you with, "Jack, the old boss, never said anything about that." Respond with, "I am not your old boss."
- She tries, "If this is so important, how is it that you never said anything about it before?" Respond with, "I thought that you would have been alert enough to take care of it without my direction."
- She claims that work is not affected. Donna responds to the charge of wasting time with, "I get my work done, don't I?" Respond with, "Yes you do, but you interfere with the work of others and set a bad example for the new employees."

3. *The Employee Counterattacks*
- She threatens to go over your head.
- She threatens to quit.
- She accuses you of the same behavior, "You have some nerve accusing me of that. I have seen you doing the very same thing many times."

If she threatens to quit, to go over your head, or to expose something damaging about you, reply that she may do whatever she chooses, but that you recommend that she give long and serious thought to such a drastic move and what impact it can have on her future.

4. *The Employee Tries to Sidetrack the Discussion*
- She blames others. "Michael does the same thing. How is it you never say anything to him?"
- She blames a myriad of personal problems at home.

If the employee tries to sidetrack the discussion, respond that nothing will be accomplished by accusing others. If she blames problems at home, channel the discussion back to the work situation. However, if signs and symptoms suggest a serious personal problem, such as drugs, alcohol, or financial distress, recommend professional help. In most instances a good comment is, "Peggy, I am not qualified to help you with those kinds of problems. I can recommend a counselor if you like, but for now let's get back to the problem of laboratory safety."

When individuals refuse to cooperate, get belligerent, clam up, or storm out of your office, they may do so because this response has worked for them in the past. If Bruce runs out of your office, do not chase after him. Simply wait until later in the day or the next day, and then send for him again. Respond to loud angry outcries with, "You are starting to yell, Andrea."

A person who suddenly clams up may be trying to decide whether or not to say something of a sensitive nature. If you break the silence too soon, you may never know what it was she wanted to say. If the silence persists, say "Leon, I thought we were having a conversation." Lean forward and look like you expect a response. If this does not work, give a sigh, and remark that it is obvious that you both are wasting time, and the meeting will have to be postponed. Reschedule, then send Leon home or back to work.

If it becomes obvious that you are not getting near a solution, do not make it a matter of wills. Simply state your position, what you expect, and then end the meeting.

Postmeeting Activities

Document the highlights of the session. Record the date, problem, employee's comments (exact words are best), the agreed-upon resolution, any warning given by you, and the deadline for acceptable response. Remember that this meeting may ultimately be the first step in a disciplinary process.

If the policy in your department is to put a copy of the report in the person's personnel file, you must give the employee a copy. It is good practice to provide such a copy even when the report is not placed in official files.

Do not discuss the meeting with anyone other than your superior or a member of the human resources department. Do not breath a sigh of relief when the meeting is over, and then fail to watch closely for developments. To do so confirms what the employee thought in the first place—that this was much ado about nothing. She will quickly revert to the old bad habit.

Follow-up Action

Monitor the subsequent behavior and take additional action if necessary. Spot changes for the better and reinforce them through praise. Identify specific concerns that call for exploration or reassurance.

If the undesired behavior or result persists, you are faced with several choices. You can extend the deadline if there has been some progress; you can institute disciplinary actions; or you can counsel again. Most often you will choose to repeat the counseling session. Now, however, you have two problems: the initial one and the new problem of the employee failing to deliver on her promise.

Your objectives in the repeat session are: (1) to let the employee know that you are aware of the continued problem; (2) to inform the employee of the risk she is taking; and (3) to give the employee one more chance before disciplinary action is taken. If you hold a repeat session, get your boss or a representative of the human resources department to sit in on the meeting. This adds to the gravity to the situation from the perspective of the employee and provides you with support.

Following are the seven key points to be covered at this session:

1. Review the agreements reached at the previous session.
2. State what you have observed or learned that indicates the agreement has been broached.
3. Ask for an explanation.
4. Insist on a new solution or effort.
5. Indicate the consequences of continued noncompliance. Avoid making a threat that you do not intend to carry out.
6. Agree on the new action to be taken and a new follow-up date.
7. Indicate your reluctance to give up on the employee and your belief that she can correct the situation.

PRINCIPLES THAT ENSURE SUCCESSFUL INTERVENTIONS

- Initially confront as a friend, not as an antagonist.
- Be direct and honest.
- Listen more than you talk.
- Say how you feel. Ask the employee how she feels.
- Select the best time and place for confrontations.
- Do not nit-pick.
- Make the employee come up with solutions.
- Go for win/win solutions.
- Be willing to compromise.
- Work with facts, not assumptions.
- Be optimistic. Expect positive results.
- Preserve the employee's self-esteem.
- Do not pontificate or be condescending.
- Do not expect the impossible.
- Look for the good in the person.

- Catch the employee doing something right and reward it.
- Monitor and reinforce.

REFERENCE

1. Umiker W. *Management Skills for the New Health Care Supervisor.* 2nd ed. Gaithersburg, Md: Aspen Publishers; 1993.

9. Disciplining Difficult Employees

Disciplining is not punishing, at least not at first. Disciplining is an educational effort to nudge unsatisfactory performance up to an acceptable level while preserving the employee's perceptions of self-worth. The initial goal is not to grease the slide toward separation. Rather, the goal is to provide traction for employees to climb back—to correct the behavior and to salvage the employee.

Disciplining usually addresses behavioral deviations rather than uncomplicated underperformance, although both can result in termination of employment. Discipline should be fair, firm, and fast. Delay only increases emotional stress—especially yours. If all you do is complain to others about an employee while doing nothing, then you deserve what you get—continued problems and loss of respect of your followers and superiors.

Today's managers are reluctant to fire people because of all the roadblocks and potential legal backlashes that may result from such action. Yate[1] notes: "It is nothing short of alarming how readily many companies will hang on to long-term substandard employees." In many organizations, employees can avoid being fired if they perform at 50% or less of their capacity. However, according to Townsend,[2] purging bad performers is as good a tonic for the organization as is rewarding the star performers. One surprising observation is that most fired people will subsequently say that it was one of the best things that ever happened to them.

Skilled discipline has been likened to a red-hot sizzling stove. It provides a warning, does not discriminate, and is immediate, consistent, and effective. Disciplinary measures are less frequently required when managers are skilled in selecting new employees, provide thorough orientation and training, address individual motivational needs, and are competent counselors. The best discipline—self-discipline—is achieved when employees are treated as responsible adults. Some managers treat their employees like children and then are surprised when these employees behave like kids. Managers who practice management by intimidation spend much of their time trying to catch people doing something wrong. The employees respond not so much by cleaning up their act as by avoiding being caught.

WHY EMPLOYEES VIOLATE RULES

There are at least nine major reasons why employees violate rules:

1. They do not know what the rules are. They have never been told the rules, never understood them, or have forgotten them.
2. They were told what the rules are, but not why the rules are needed.
3. They perceive the rules as meaningless or unnecessarily restrictive.
4. They do not think the rules apply to them. This is especially true of some administrative and professional employees.
5. They see others, especially their superiors, violating the rules.
6. They perceive the risk or penalties of rule violations to be less than the advantages or pleasures involved.
7. They misbehave to get attention or to retaliate against perceived wrongs.
8. They have a drug, alcohol, or psychiatric problem.
9. They are misfits, malcontents, or criminals.

EMPLOYEE REACTIONS TO BEING DISCIPLINED

1. They quit and leave.
2. They "quit" and stay because of vested time, unwillingness to change jobs or life-style, or lack of opportunities elsewhere.
3. They seek redress via unions, courts, the Equal Employment Opportunity Commission (EEOC), the Occupational Safety and Health Administration (OSHA), or other governmental agencies. A significant percentage of employees who are disciplined resort to filing complaints or grievances.

A BASIC PRINCIPLE OF DISCIPLINE

Appropriate discipline operates on a reward/penalty ratio. When an employee knowingly violates a rule, he consciously or subconsciously believes that the reward is greater than the penalty (or the risk). Our goal as managers is to recognize the "reward" that the employee perceives, to reduce its value, to increase the penalty, or both.

PROGRESSIVE DISCIPLINE

This system of discipline is called "progressive" because it implies that the disciplinary measures will progress to a resolution of the problem. In its traditional form, progressive discipline consists of the following steps:

1. The oral reprimand
2. The written reprimand
3. Suspension
4. Discharge

Of course, other disciplinary actions are available, such as withholding of salary raises, bonuses, or promotions, giving a lower performance rating, placing the employee on probation, and demoting or denying special requests for educational support, time off, or other special benefits.

Serious offenses are subject to immediate dismissal, but most must move through one or more of the other stages. Organizations should provide lists of common violations and what penalties are appropriate for each.

The Oral Reprimand

When giving an oral reprimand, use the same counseling technique that was recommended in the previous chapter. Since that counseling has now escalated to disciplining, however, you are less empathetic, more distant, and more formal. Omit any social talk before getting into the discussion. The employee should get the impression that your patience is running out. For example:

"Jason, your previous attempt at improving your performance has not worked, and I cannot tolerate any more of this behavior. Let's get back to the drawing board." Insist on finishing what you have to say. If he tries to interrupt, say "Jason, please let me finish." Insert a positive note: "This is way below what you are capable of, Jason. In fact, I still have difficulty understanding it." Now give Jason air time, but cut it off when he starts to repeat or tries to divert your attention to something or someone else. Bring him back to the issue with, "Jason, we are here to discuss your problem. Let's stick to that." Warn of future action: "Jason, if this is not corrected immediately, it will be necessary for me to (specify a punishment)."

Listen for a big sigh—the venting.[3] The sigh occurs when the person is ready to rationalize and to try to solve the problem. Collaborate in assisting the person to come up with a new solution or a new affirmation. Insist on a commitment. After the meeting, treat the person in a friendly fashion as you did after a counseling session. You and the employee have joined forces against a common enemy. You are allies in the endeavor.

The Written Reprimand

In a high percentage of cases, the written reprimand ultimately leads to a separation—voluntary or otherwise—so proceed with caution. Your human resources department may have a special form that you must use for this purpose. Discuss the problem with your boss or a member of the human resources department before you write up the report.

When you meet with the employee, explain that a written reprimand constitutes a formal warning and will be documented in his personnel file. Review the previous counseling sessions for the same problem. Be specific as to your expectations and the final date for compliance (eg, "If within the next 60 days you are late for work one more time without an acceptable excuse, you will be sent home on a one-day suspension without pay"). Insist that the employee read and sign the report. Inform him of the right to attach a rebuttal or to confer with your superior.

Basic Components of a Written Disciplinary Warning
1. Description of the problem: state facts, not assumptions, hearsay, or opinion; give dates if possible; record names of witnesses and/or involved persons.
2. Record of previous warnings: give dates; indicate what conclusions and solutions were reached; record what changes in conduct, if any, resulted.
3. Record of previous written reprimands or punitive actions: attach copies; indicate what punitive measures had been imposed; state what changes in conduct, if any, resulted.
4. The employee's explanation, denial, or rebuttal: if employee chooses this option, include a copy of it; if employee chooses not to document this, describe what the employee stated, as accurately as possible, and include a statement that the employee chose not to prepare a document.
5. Record of punitive action now being decreed: include deadline date; describe exactly what will not be tolerated; include a statement that the punishment was explained to the employee and that the employee understood what was stated; affix your signature and ask the employee to sign; if the employee refuses to

sign, call in a witness, repeat the process, and have the witness sign attesting to the employee's refusal to sign the report.

6. Statute of limitations: After a period of time (eg, six months) without further incidents, remove the record from the person's file (tell him that that is what you will do).

Suspensions

Some offenses call for immediate suspension or discharge. The list of causes for immediate dismissal varies from employer to employer. Fighting on the job, theft, unethical behavior, unauthorized release of patient information, falsifying reports, or use of illegal drugs are examples of behaviors that usually call for immediate firing. In these situations, there may have been no previous oral or written reprimands. If the employee has received oral and written warnings in the past, it may not be necessary to hold a formal meeting. The suspension document should be prepared carefully and given directly to the employee by you. Your human resources department will provide you with the necessary form or give you instructions on how to prepare the report. You may be asked to submit a detailed report, and the human resources department will prepare the official document. When the employee returns to work, treat him like you would any other employee.

Discharge

The prescribed procedure for discharge, both process and content, must be adhered to carefully. Make certain that you have the authority to carry the disciplinary process this far. If possible, have the discharge implemented by the human resources department. To sustain a discharge against legal challenges, you must be able to prove the following:

1. That what you alleged did take place, involved the employee, and warrants the discharge.
2. That such behavior has not been condoned in the past, or that others have been disciplined for similar offenses.
3. The sequence of progressive discipline followed prescribed policy and procedures.
4. The employee made no genuine effort to heed the previous warnings, even though he had been informed as to the consequences.
5. The firing was based on behavior or results, not on any of the following (which fall under the category of "wrongful discharge"): employee whistleblowing regarding lack of occupational safety or unethical or illegal activities by management or condoned by

managers; employee charges of sexual harassment; employee called to jury or military duty; employee claims for worker's compensation; employee engagement in prounion activities; employee filing grievances regarding breached promises of permanent work, salary increase, or promotion ("implied contract").

DOCUMENTATION OF DISCIPLINARY ACTION

Carefully follow the procedure for documentation as prescribed by your organization. The first sentence usually states what action is being taken and what caused the need for discipline.[4] For example: "Beginning on Monday, February 12, you are placed on three-day suspension without pay for excessive tardiness at the beginning of workdays." (Note: the word "excessive" must be defined according to company policy.) This is followed by a brief description of the precipitating incident (eg, "This action is prompted by your arrival at 0900—60 minutes late—on Friday, February 9, after three previous verbal warnings and one written reprimand"). Finally, state what will happen if the situation is not corrected (eg, "Additional tardiness will result in termination"). Conclude with a clear statement of any time period imposed (eg, "Your progress will be reviewed again on May 1").

THE TERMINATION MEETING

A termination interview should never be initiated with a possibility of reconsideration in mind. All such possibilities should have been exhausted before the final meeting. The simplest and best agenda goes something like this:

"Greg, you have received your discharge notice, right? Greg, I am sorry things have not worked out. Here is your final paycheck, plus severance pay, unused vacation, and sick leave time. Good luck, Greg."

NONPUNITIVE DISCIPLINE

Punishment breeds resistance, encourages subterfuge, and undermines an employee's willingness to make future contributions to the organization. The nonpunitive or "positive" disciplinary approach has been successful in overcoming many of these adverse effects.[5]

With the nonpunitive approach, the employee is treated as a person who has difficulty complying with your performance expectations. Encouragement replaces threats. Rules are referred to as employee responsibilities, while verbal and written warnings are expressed as suggestions.

Discussions are low key, with emphasis on problem solving. John is told that his present performance threatens the organization's success and his future with the organization. The suggestion is made that there is a poor employee-job fit and that a change in employment may be beneficial for all parties.

The most radical departure from the traditional disciplinary approach is the one-day suspension with pay. The employee is given a "day of decision." The supervisor says something like the following:

"John, our solutions have not worked. I have serious concerns about whether you want to continue here. John, I do not want a commitment right now. Take the rest of the day (or tomorrow) to think over what you want to do; then let me know what you have decided. If you want to continue as a member of our team—fine. However, you will have to give me a signed, firm commitment that you will fulfill all your responsibilities. If you do not, then we both have failed and your employment will end. As a token of our faith in you, and as a sign that we want you to stay with us, you will receive full pay for the day."[5]

An employer may insist that an employee who elects to stay must document the proposed solution and sign it (eg, "I affirm my desire to fulfill my responsibility to.... I understand that if I... [or if I do not...] I will be terminating my employment here").

This strategy has: (1) reduced the filing of grievances over terminations; (2) decreased involuntary turnover; and (3) improved morale. The only objections have been from the employee's coworkers who resent someone getting a day off with pay while they must do that employee's work.

SUGGESTIONS FOR BETTER DISCIPLINARY ACTIONS

Know:

- Exactly what the unacceptable behavior is and what policy or rule has been violated.
- Mitigating circumstances.
- The scope of your authority.
- How similar offenses have been handled in the past.

Assume:

- The employee wants to be a good performer.
- The employee perceives some benefit from his unacceptable behavior.
- You or others may be partly to blame.
- You have many options, including probation, holding up the next pay raise, unfavorable comments on the next performance review, denying special requests, and awarding less pleasant assignments.
- Across-the-board salary increases for poor performers are counter-productive.

Act:

- Consult with your superior or the human resources department.
- Act quickly once you have the information you need.
- Be consistent and fair.
- Use punishment only as a last resort.
- Talk to the employee in private.
- Select penalties that are appropriate for the offenses.
- Document, document, document.
- When you discipline an employee who is popular with his coworkers, you must rely on the support you have built up with your team; if they trust you, they will support any decision you make that they regard as fair.

Do Not:

- Let misbehavior develop into habits.
- Act before you get the facts.
- Be apologetic; it decreases the effectiveness of the warning.
- Use words like loyalty, attitude, work ethic, professionalism, or maturity.
- Say "Management expects..."; do say "I expect...."
- Trap yourself into a series of verbal warnings for the same problem with the same employee; discipline must escalate.
- Request that the employee think about how bad his behavior has been; instead, ask him to reflect on how good things were when he performed well.

REFERENCES

1. Yate M. *Keeping the Best*. Holbrook, Mass: Bob Adams Inc; 1991.
2. Townsend R. *Up the Organization*. New York, NY: Fawcett World Library; 1971.
3. Sherman VC. *From Losers to Winners*. New York, NY: Nightingale-Conant Corp; 1987.
4. Jonker P, Reeves TZ. The hidden messages in disciplinary memos. *Supervis Manage*. 1991;36:4-5.
5. Redeker JR. Discipline, II: the nonpunitive approach works by design. *Personnel*. 1985;62:7-10.

10. Conflict Resolution and Confrontation

Conflict is not all bad. It can move people to take a second look at situations, lead to service improvements, and enhance future interpersonal relationships if handled expertly. In the two previous chapters, we discussed behavioral problems of subordinates—individuals who either had to straighten up or risk being discharged. Supervisors also often find themselves embroiled in conflicts with superiors, peers, and internal or external customers or suppliers. Sometimes the conflict is interdepartmental rather than interpersonal, and within a department or other unit disagreements may occur between work groups. In other instances, the attitudes or behaviors of the people who report to us leave something to be desired but fall into the category of annoyances rather than acts that are amenable to counseling or disciplining. Misunderstandings, disagreements, conflicts, and confrontations also arise between friends and close associates—none of whom could be called "difficult people."

In this chapter and the next, we offer some generic yet practical advice for dealing with interpersonal conflicts of any nature before focusing on the various forms of difficult people.

MAJOR CAUSES OF CONFLICT

1. Unclear Expectations

Subordinates may not know what they are supposed to do, how it is to be done, and how good the results must be. Policies and rules may be ambiguous. Then there are always people who assume that they are exempt from the rules.

2. Garbled Communication

In chapter 2 we discussed communication barriers, perceptions, assumptions, and other causes of communication breakdowns. Any of these can result in misunderstandings and conflicts and even lead to the filing of grievances. We can all cite examples of hurt feelings and broken friendships that resulted from distortions or frank untruths that get into our corporate "grapevine" and behave like a computer virus. Many of us must admit that we have offended others and may have made fools of ourselves by taking action or making statements based on erroneous information.

3. Hierarchical Conflicts

Disputes between the various management levels may occur as hospital administrations become more complex. For example, a PhD or MD may resent taking orders from a young MBA manager.

4. Incompatibilities or Disagreements

Differences of value systems, goals, temperaments, attitudes, or ethics often produce difficulties in the workplace. These are often complex, with overlays of race, religion, nationality, age, politics, sense of humor, and general likes and dislikes.

5. Resource Allocation

These conflicts may be over funds, space, time, personnel, or equipment. Time conflicts may be over staffing schedules, especially for nights, holidays, or weekends. Such conflicts may occur between individual people or between larger departments.

6. Competition for Power

Power struggles often arise because authority is not spelled out in position descriptions or organizational charts. For example, the technical director and the medical director of a laboratory may engage in bitter power disputes.

7. Operational or Staffing Changes

Changes in processes, systems, workflows, or protocols affect interpersonal relationships, and anything that impacts these relationships carries a potential for conflict. Likewise, changes in assignments, work shifts, workstations, or schedules are common causes of disagreements.

The etiology of conflict is not always apparent. Often a covert issue is hidden by a less important overt factor. Other situations may become murky because the actual cause of the conflict is multifactorial.

GOALS AND OBJECTIVES OF CONFLICT RESOLUTION

The proactive goal of conflict resolution is to prevent conflicts from ever occurring in the first place. When that is not possible, you should opt to keep small conflicts from growing into big ones. To do so, you will have to hone your conflict resolution abilities. The objectives of such confrontations include diffusing anger, venting feelings, and converting conflicts into problem solving exercises.

BASIC STRATEGIES OF CONFLICT CONFRONTATION

Each of the following strategies is appropriate for certain situations. The trick is to pick the right strategy for the right situation.

Avoid

Avoidance may include denying that a problem exists, physically escaping, or passing the buck. Such procrastination may lead to sleepless nights or augment feelings of guilt. The major hazard is that the problem remains unresolved. Anger builds and later explodes. In some instances, however, avoidance is the best solution.

This strategy is appropriate when:

- It is not your problem.
- There is nothing you can do about it.
- It is not important.
- Additional information is needed.
- You or the other individual is emotionally upset.
- Potential disruption outweighs the benefits of resolution.
- The situation will probably ameliorate if you can wait it out.

Fight

Several booby traps are hidden in this "do it my way or else" approach. For one thing, you can lose. And even if you win, your opponents may regroup, return to the fray, and wait for another opportunity to retaliate or become saboteurs. At times, however, you may have to lay down the law.

This strategy is appropriate when:

- Quick action is needed (eg, life-threatening situations); you do not convene a committee when a fire breaks out.
- Certain rules must be enforced, such as safety regulations.
- Ethical or legal issues are involved.
- Nothing else works.

Surrender

Surrender involves conceding or accommodating—"Okay, okay, I will do it." The nonassertive person succumbs to this in almost every conflict, thus building up internal frustration as self-esteem erodes. But in some instances, even the most assertive individual must wave the white flag.

This strategy is appropriate when:

- You are wrong.
- It does not matter to you but is important to them.
- You have little or no chance to win.
- Harmony and stability are especially important.
- Giving in on a minor item means winning a more important one later.

Compromise

You must often settle for this partial-win strategy. Compromise permits each party to get part of what they want, so that both parties share some satisfaction (and some dissatisfaction). Most union/management disputes are settled in this manner.

On the negative side, neither party gets everything they want. In addition, compromise may involve game playing, with each side pumping up its demands or disguising them. A common error is to adopt this alternative prematurely, without making a greater effort at collaboration.

This strategy is appropriate when:

- Opposing goals are incompatible.
- A temporary settlement to complex issues is needed.
- Time constraints call for an expedient solution.

The following introduction to negotiating dialogues is recommended by Bernstein and Rozen[1]:

"As I understand it, you want...and I want...."
"I am willing to...if you are willing to...."

After agreement has been reached, the compromise is spelled out very clearly. For example: "So, we have agreed that you will let us use your conference room on Mondays and Fridays. In return, we will keep the audiovisual equipment in good working condition."

Collaborate

Collaboration is working together to find solutions that satisfy both parties. This win/win approach is usually the best alternative, but it often requires a creative solution because the best answer is one that neither side originally considered.

This approach consists of turning conflict between individuals into a mutual attack on the problem. For example: "How can we solve this in a way that satisfies both of us?" A great strength of this approach is that it builds positive relationships.[2] Weaknesses of the method are the length of time often required, possible delayed decisions, and even frustration when no consensus is reached.

This strategy is appropriate when:

- The issue is too important to be settled any other way.
- Commitment is sought via a consensus.
- Different perspectives are to be explored.

PREPARATIONS FOR A CONFLICT RESOLUTION

What we are calling conflict resolution, others (attorneys, purchasing agents, union officials, and diplomats) call negotiating. Whatever the term, planning is essential when preparing to confront a conflict and, in the long run, it saves time. The planning process consists of two steps: analysis and strategy.

Analysis

Diagnose the situation by asking yourself:

- What are the facts?
- What is the cause of the conflict?

- What are likely to be the points of agreement and disagreement?
- What do you want to accomplish?
- What are your minimal acceptable results?
- What do you think the other party wants?
- What are the strengths and weaknesses of your stance?
- What false assumptions or incorrect perceptions might the other person have?

The answers you get to these questions help you to determine which strategy to use and also make you better prepared to handle the situation.

Strategy

First, based on your analysis, select a basic strategy (see previous list). You may be able to avoid the confrontation, but this is usually a poor choice. You always have the option of breaking off an encounter at any step of the way.

When you must face an aggressive person or situation, first prepare yourself for the encounter. Then make your move—do not procrastinate. The longer you respond to another person in a passive manner, the more difficult it is to change to an assertive style. Prepare the arguments you can make to maximize the value of positive aspects, to minimize the negatives, and to counter the other person's arguments.

THE THREE KEYS TO ASSERTIVE CONFRONTATIONS

1. Success Imagery

This consists of visualizing a successful confrontation. You picture your body language, hear your words and voice tone, and envision a successful outcome. Athletes and professional speakers have used this technique with great success for years.

2. Self-talk

Self-talk is simply converting negative thoughts to positive ones when talking to oneself. All of us carry on inner dialogues with ourselves all day long. When we are in a passive mode or when our self-esteem is low, these internal conversations are negative and pessimistic. Our subconscious mind conjures up statements like, "I could never say that" or "She will just blow me away."

Let your positive affirmations take control. Say to yourself, "I will be in control." Avoid weak statements like, "I am going to try to stand up to her next time." Instead, use rational assertions to address your concerns. For example, Supervisor Jane is preparing for a performance appraisal interview with Joe, a marginal performer who always responds angrily to any criticism:

> Jane's concern: "As soon as I give him his rating he is going to get red in the face and start shouting."
> Rational assertion: "I can put up with that. It never lasts long. I will just lean forward and stay silent."
> Jane's concern: "He will get up, storm out of my office, and go around complaining about me."
> Rational assertion: "The others are fed up with his immature behavior. He will get no support from them."
> Jane's concern: "He will resign."
> Rational assertion: "He often threatens to do that but never has—and maybe we would be better off without him."

3. Rehearsing

After you have selected your dialogue and the appropriate body language, rehearse the anticipated encounter over and over. Do it in front of a mirror. Verbalize out loud. Still better, get a friend or relative to role-play with you. Do not be satisfied until your performance is down pat.

THE OPPOSING FORCES ARE ENGAGED, NOW WHAT?

After outlining the problem, focus on areas of agreement. For example: "Lynn, I think we agree that we both want what is best for our patients, right?"

Use the strategy of salespeople who ask a series of questions, each of which they know will be answered with a "yes." It is then easier to get a yes to a more controversial question that follows this sequence.

Be an attentive listener, keying in on what the other person is saying. Do not be guilty of "mindscripting," which is switching your attention from what the other person is saying to thinking about what you want to say next. Be empathetic. Respect the other person's feelings, but still feel free to respond in a manner of your choosing.

Let the person know that you hear and understand. Validate her response with something like, "As I understand it, Joan, you are angry because I asked one of your assistants to give me a hand with my project. Is that right?" Validating has two benefits. It clarifies the problem and lets the person know that what she is saying is important.

Shoot for a solution that satisfies both of you. Often it pays to ask exactly what it is that the person wants. An angry person may have to stop and think about it, or you may find that what she wanted is actually less than what you were prepared to offer. On the other hand, do not neglect to say what it is that you want. You may be pleasantly surprised by the response.

Keep things in perspective. People tend to exaggerate when they are upset. This increases anxiety and makes problem solving more difficult. When verbally cornered, say "You are making me uncomfortable." The person will usually back off immediately or even get derailed. If you feel your heart pounding, face turning red, voice rising, and fists clenching, call a time out. Do not worry about what excuse you use. For example: "I need a little time to collect my thoughts, Alice," or "I find myself getting upset, Steve. Let's take a ten-minute break, okay?"

To avoid retaliation, use the "strawperson" technique. This is a way of expressing your opinion indirectly. It is most appropriate when dealing with a strongly opinionated boss or a know-it-all. Instead of saying, "Dr. John, I think you are wrong," say, "Dr. John, how would you respond to a laboratorian who claims that no better tests are available for diagnosing that disease?" Dr. John will suspect what you are doing, but if she retaliates, it will have to be against the unnamed "laboratorian" and not against you.

CONFRONTING AN ANGRY PERSON

Anger, which is a physiological response, should be differentiated from hostility, which is a state of mind, and aggressiveness, which is a behavior. An outburst of anger often represents the accumulation of a series of frustrations, fears, guilts, or other emotions. The precipitating factor may not be the most important causative agent.[3] In chapter 4, we discussed how to cope with our own anger, and later we will focus on some specific kinds of hostile people. At this point, however, let's look at some general aspects of confronting angry people.

People are more likely to express anger toward those who have less power. Sales representatives, service providers, spouses, children, and pets take more than their fair share of abuse. Anger is manifested by bitter sarcasm, accusations, crying, sulking, pouting, and walking away (often accompanied by door slamming and angry words). Yells, threats, or physical attacks are, of course, more frightening.

We may provoke anger in others when we criticize, pressure, threaten, deny, irritate, or deride—anything that attacks self-esteem. Almost anyone can be provoked into anger if the stimulus is intense enough, but each of us has a different threshold. Some subordinates and associates are super-sensitive. They may have explosive tempers on very short fuses. Some use anger to get out of unpleasant assignments. These individuals take everything personally and quickly and angrily charge favoritism or discrimination when things do not go their way.

You seldom can change these people, but you can modify your response to their behavior. Focus on your goal. Do not argue, just press your demand. Say, "I know you are angry about this, but when can you start what I just asked you to do?"

The Three Essentials for Controlling a Potentially Explosive Situation

1. The person who speaks first CONTROLS THE MOOD.
2. The person who asks the most questions CONTROLS THE DIRECTION.
3. The person who listens best CONTROLS THE OUTCOME.

Using these essentials, here are some tips for handling an angry physician or other customer who walks into your office:

1. If you sense anger, get up and out from behind your desk. Move toward the person, but no closer than 6 to 7 feet.
2. Speak first and softly. Greet the person and ask how you can help.
3. Listen until she runs out of gas. Do not interrupt.
4. Play back the facts you have heard, and state how you interpret her feelings.
5. Offer explanations without excuses. Do not blame other people, computers, policies, or workloads. Anger subsides with offers of help, not alibis.
6. Offer a solution. Bargain if necessary.
7. Thank the person for alerting you to the situation.

Tips for More Effective Confrontation

1. Be prepared, just as you would be for a debate.
2. Pick the best time and place. Do not meet when your self-esteem is low or when either of you is upset.
3. Regard the other person not as an enemy but as a partner in problem solving.
4. Clarify the other person's viewpoint, and yours. Do not proceed until these viewpoints and desired outcomes are crystal clear. Do an audible perception check by paraphrasing what the person said: "Do I hear you saying that...?"

5. Focus first on a point of agreement and work from there.
6. Be assertive but not aggressive. Use short responses, which are more assertive. Longer ones suggest passivity or aggressiveness.
7. Attack the problem, not the other person.
8. Do not cause the opponent to lose face. Do not threaten or issue ultimatums.
9. Do not be sarcastic or critical.
10. To avoid retaliation, use the "strawperson" technique.
11. Watch your body language. Maintain eye contact, sit or stand up straight, and appear relaxed. Do not fidget or squirm. Avoid threatening gestures such as fingerpointing, clenched fists, crossed arms, hands on hips, or scowling. Smile when you agree; remain expressionless when you disagree.
12. Control your voice. Keep its volume, pitch, and rate under control. Stop if you find it growing louder, faster, or at a higher pitch.
13. Be diplomatic and tentative when facing firm resistance. Use words like "maybe," "perhaps," or "you may be right."
14. When verbally cornered or upset, escape by pleading stress.
15. Do not get stuck believing that your solution is the only good one. Focus on the benefits to the other person.
16. Propose incentives for collaboration: "If you…, then I will…."
17. End on a positive note.

REFERENCES

1. Bernstein AJ, Rozen SC. *Dinosaur Brains: Dealing With All Those Impossible People at Work*. New York, NY: John Wiley & Sons; 1989.

2. Kirby T. *The Can-do Manager: How to Get Your Employees to Take Risks, Take Action, and Get Things Done*. New York, NY: AMACOM; 1989.

3. Tavris C. *Anger: The Misunderstood Emotion*. New York, NY: Simon & Schuster; 1982.

11. Principles of Coping With Difficult People

The old cliché "different strokes for different folks" is true. Each different kind of difficult person requires a different remedial approach. In fact, within a single category—hostile people, for example—there are many subsets of people, each of whom responds somewhat differently to various coping methods. That is why coping with difficult people is so difficult.

Nevertheless, we can use certain general principles. Rather than repeat these tidbits in each subsequent chapter, we have elected to group them within this chapter. Like all universal tools or techniques, they are not as effective as measures that are designed for specific purposes, yet they do provide a good overview.

THE THREE MAJOR KINDS OF PROBLEMS

1. Performance that does not meet expectations.
2. Behavior that violates rules, policies, or ethics.
3. Employees who are unable to get along with other people.

When employees exhibit these behaviors, who really has the problem? You, the supervisor, do! Employees who are working at 50% efficiency do not think they have a problem. They get paid each day and have a lot of energy left over when they take off for home. If difficult people thought that they had problems, they would change what they were doing or not doing. One of the reasons that managers fail to change problem behavior is that they do not convince the difficult people that they have a problem. Why do difficult people treat others like they do? Tucker[1] offers these reasons:

- They do not trust their leaders or others.
- They think that others are too demanding (conceited, manipulative, untrustworthy, etc).
- They are jealous.
- They consider others, especially their superiors, as undeserving of their support.
- They feel neglected or unappreciated.
- They are more impressed by other employers or colleagues.
- They think they can get away with it.
- They know that their leaders can be bluffed.
- They think others will support them or not support their leaders.
- They think they are indispensable.
- They think they can blackmail their superiors.

THE THREE CRITICAL MISTAKES MADE BY SUPERVISORS

When managers are faced with problem behavior, they may respond incorrectly in one of the three following ways:

1. They do nothing or wait too long before they act. Many managers are reluctant to tell an employee what they do not like.
2. They incorrectly ascribe the deviant behavior to "bad attitude" or "poor work ethic."
3. They "gunnysack," saving up all the problems and then exploding at a later date, often in response to some trivial transgression.

Why Supervisors Fail to Take Remedial Measures

- They do not know what is going on.
- They ignore it because they:
    think it is unimportant.
    fear they are on shaky grounds or are guilty of the same thing.
    are afraid of the person or of how that person will react.
    are afraid that a valued employee may quit.
    assume the situation will self-correct or someone else will take care of it.
    decide to wait until the next performance appraisal.
    do not know how to conduct counseling interviews or have had unpleasant previous experiences with them.

POOR ATTITUDE IS NOT A MAJOR CAUSE
OF POOR PERFORMANCE

Probably a minority of behavioral problems are attitudinal. Poor attitude is believed to be such a common cause of problems because it is easy to claim and it takes the blame off the leaders.

More often employees do not:

■ Know what they are expected to do. Position descriptions, orientation programs, training, and coaching are inadequate. Personnel handbooks are substituted for person-to-person indoctrination.

■ Know how well they must perform. Work standards are not provided.

■ Have the necessary education or skills when first hired, and they are not given on-the-job training.

■ Know how they are performing. The necessary feedback is missing.

■ Get rewarded when they do well. Negative consequences follow good performance. Coworkers make fun of their efforts, or supervisors load them down with additional work. Poor performers, on the other hand, are rewarded for substandard performance by having their workload reduced, or they get more attention from their supervisor (negative strokes are better than no strokes).

"IT IS ALL JUST USING COMMON SENSE"

How often have you heard this? If this were true, we must not have many managers with common sense, because innumerable persistent behavioral problems drive supervisors up the walls. How effective are "common sense" solutions for the following situations:

■ We tell our son to clean up his room or else.
■ We tell a patient not to worry about a diagnostic procedure about to be performed.
■ We tell a departing guest to drive carefully.
■ We tell two feuding subordinates to shake hands and stop bickering.
■ We hold still another counseling session with an employee who is habitually late.

Watzlawick and associates[2] point out that effective solutions often violate the tenets of common sense. They believe that creativity often succeeds when logic fails. For example, they claim that insomniacs are more likely to fall asleep if they keep their eyes wide open and try to stay awake.

FOUR PROBLEM SOLVING STRATEGIES

1. Avoid the Problem ("Wait and See")

The problem may not be important enough to merit your immediate attention. It may be a transient or self-correcting situation or is not in your sphere of responsibility. For example:

- A new cytotechnologist complains about new productivity (screening) levels.
- A subordinate is in the grieving phase of a family member's death.

2. Apply Symptomatic Measures ("Quick Fix")

These are temporary solutions to situations that demand immediate action. The resolution of the basic problem is postponed or may not require subsequent additional action. For example:

- Two angry employees are on the verge of coming to blows. You send them both home. The next day you start investigating the problem.
- A phlebotomist punctures his finger as a result of negligence. You escort him to the emergency room for treatment. Later you review the proper protocol with him.

3. Change Policy, Procedure, or Assignment ("New Ground Rules")

What the person did, or did not do, is no longer a violation or a deficiency. For example:

- The dress code is liberalized. Employees are no longer cited for beards or long hair.
- Absenteeism is redefined. The number of allowable days is increased.

4. Undertake a Comprehensive Investigation and Resolution ("Going for Broke")

This obviously requires much more time, know-how, and savoir-faire. For example:

- It is reported that "someone" from your department is falsifying laboratory reports. You must discover who the person is.

■ An employee files a sexual harassment grievance. You must interview both parties and reach a resolution.

HOW TO ANALYZE A PROBLEM

1. Define the problem in concrete terms, then determine if it is important enough to do something about. How does it affect work performance, the difficult people's coworkers, and you? Document these effects. You may need these later to support a decision to discipline or to counter a grievance or other legal action. Omit opinions, conjectures, and diagnoses. Record only objective evidence. Later on, when you counsel the difficult person, read parts of this to him. The fact that it is documented will help to convince the person that the problem is a serious one. If you have difficulty defining and delineating the problem, you probably do not have a significant problem, or it is one you should be able to live with it. Celebrate!

2. Review the remedial measures that have been tried and how effective they were. If they did not work, determine what went wrong.

3. Determine exactly what you want to achieve:
"To improve Leslie's attendance" (too vague).
"Leslie's average absences are not to exceed the department's average—one day/month. Her Monday attendance is not to exceed that of other days of the week" (good).

4. Study the reward/risk ratio. What benefits of this behavior may be perceived by Leslie (eg, time for taking care of personal matters, extra sleep, or getting rides to work)? What risks are incurred (eg, chewed out by boss, nasty remarks from colleagues, work piling up on desk, or poor performance rating)?

5. Brainstorm as many alternative solutions as possible. Ideally, the solution comes from the difficult person and meets your approval. Solicit input from your boss, your human resources department, or a professional advisor.

SIGNIFICANT FACTORS IN BEHAVIORAL MODIFICATION

1. Positive Reinforcement

This is catching people doing something right and rewarding them with praise and other signs of recognition. It is the most effective modality for achieving desired behavior.

Watch your difficult people for something you can praise. It does not have to be something major. Say exactly what it was that you liked. Remark how good you feel about it and do not be discouraged if the person responds with a downer such as, "Oh, do I get a raise?" or "Now what are you buttering me up for?" Just smile, shake hands, and leave.

2. Negative Reinforcement

This can be either ignoring unwanted behavior or criticizing it. People usually prefer to be reprimanded than to be ignored. Difficult people who receive little or no attention may purposely act up to get attention, just as children often do. Negative strokes are better than no strokes.

Some employees are so consistently average that they receive neither praise nor criticism, but these "old-faithfuls" should not be overlooked. Supervisors have a tendency to spend much time with their star performers and with their difficult people, while ignoring the quiet, dependable, but unspectacular workers. Then they are surprised and hurt when a loyal employee who has been taken for granted for years suddenly starts acting out.

3. Managerial Skills

The skills of motivation, communication, coaching, delegation, counseling, and career development bring out the best in people. If a supervisor does not master these skills, difficult people will spring up like dandelions.

4. Proper Tactics

Sometimes you are using the best strategy, but not the best tactics. Review your technique for positive and negative reinforcement. How do you praise good behavior and redirect negative behavior? Perhaps you need the assistance of others in your efforts. Here are three modifications to try before scrapping your game plan.

1. Have your boss sit in on the next counseling session with the recalcitrant difficult person. This shows the difficult person that you are dead serious.
2. Solicit the help of the difficult person's mentor, counselor, or a close friend. Ask them to "talk some sense" into the difficult person.
3. Gather the difficult person's family members and friends and have a grand confrontation. This technique has been very successful

in coping with individuals who have an alcohol or drug problem. The members of such groups reaffirm their love and support for the difficult person and express the fervent hope that the person will make the necessary adjustments.

A caveat: Reserve the last two options for desperate cases. They can backfire.

WHAT IF NOTHING WORKS?

Do not give up without giving each approach a stout try. You must be as determined to achieve a change as the difficult person is to wear you down and revert to his former behavioral patterns.[1]

More often than we would like to admit, all attempts to modify the behavior and attitude of difficult people fail, and we are faced with a tough choice. Should we accept and tolerate the difficult person or should we fire him? The threat of firing sometimes has the desired effect. This is especially true when dealing with alcoholics who fear the loss of the means for buying their alcohol.

Lou Holtz, Notre Dame's football coach, when asked how he handles a problem staff member replied: "If there is a problem I cannot solve, I may have to learn to live with it. If I cannot change it and I cannot live with it, I will have to divorce myself from it. My job then is to help that person find out if he might be happier elsewhere."[3]

If you decide to live with the situation, you must take measures to increase your ability to do so. Refer to the sections in chapter 4 on stress management. In extreme situations, you may need professional counseling. If you decide to fire the employee, take the appropriate action without delay. Refer to chapter 9.

PSYCHOLOGICAL GAMES: AVOID THEM IF YOU CAN

Berne[4] describes dozens of negative psychological transactions that he called "games." These are far from fun games; they are one-on-one dialogues that have as their purpose to make other people feel "not okay" or to get attention, even when that attention is negative. These games erode self-esteem and inhibit healthy rapport.

Difficult people frequently play these games. If we hope to cope with them, we must either avoid the games or abort them before they reach their usual payoffs. We must also guard against initiating such games ourselves. In these games, a socially acceptable statement that is a façade or a lie is followed by ones in which the hidden agenda is revealed—to the chagrin of the victim.

Games That Suggest The Other Person is "Not Okay"

Gotcha

> Boss (at department meeting): "Eric please document the minutes for my signature."
>
> Eric: "But I thought Laura, our secretary, was here to do that."
>
> Boss: "The discussions are too technical for Laura."
>
> Eric (three days later): "Here are the minutes."
>
> Boss: "You must have been asleep during that meeting. You missed the most important points. You also made a lot of typos, and I wanted the minutes two days ago. I guess I just can't depend on you, Eric."
>
> Analysis: The boss dislikes Eric and uses this opportunity to trap him into tackling something that the boss knows he will not be able to do well. He then takes the opportunity to blast poor Eric.

See What You Made Me Do

> Staff Nurse: "I cannot get anyone to chair that new committee."
>
> Nurse Supervisor: "Why not rotate the chair?"
>
> Staff Nurse (later): "I did what you suggested. Now things are worse. The person whose turn it is to chair the meeting usually calls in sick."
>
> Analysis: An unpopular decision is needed, and the staff nurse passes the buck to her supervisor who then is shown up as an incompetent leader—"not okay."

Yes But

> Radiology Tech: "In a nutshell, that is my problem. What should I do?"
>
> Supervisor: "Why don't you...?"
>
> Tech: "That will not work because...."
>
> Supervisor: "Have you tried...?"
>
> Tech: "Yes, but it got everybody upset."
>
> Supervisor: "I think you could...."
>
> Tech: "Yes, but that would mean coming in this weekend."
>
> Analysis: The supervisor is put down because he cannot come up with an acceptable solution. This game is closely related to SEE WHAT YOU MADE ME DO.

Games That Invite Attention by Assuming the Role of a Victim

Kick Me

> Night Laboratory Technologist: "Do not get upset, but the night nursing supervisor is going to complain about how slow I was last night."

Laboratory Supervisor: "We are getting a lot of these complaints when you are on duty."

Laboratory Technologist: "There you go picking on me again."

Analysis: Although the employee says, "Do not get upset with me," he is really inviting the supervisor to do just that. In fact, if that does not get a rise out of the supervisor, he will look for even more provocative stimuli.

In a closely related game, SCHLEMIEL, the first player commits a series of errors or clumsy acts such as spilling or dropping things and then apologizing profusely. The second player must choose between getting angry or suffering in silence. In either instance, the first player gets the payoff.

Wooden Leg

Chemistry Supervisor: "You forgot to put the contaminated glassware in the right container again."

Lab Aide: "What do you expect from a high school dropout?"

Chemistry Supervisor: "I expect you to learn simple things like that. You also neglected to clean up the tabletops."

Lab Aide: "I have only been here a few weeks."

Analysis: The employee assumes the role of victim. He takes full advantage of any excuse for not doing all that is expected of him. This is the easiest way to avoid assuming responsibility.

Games That Attempt to Divert Attention From One's Own Deficiencies by Criticizing Others

Blemish

ER Physician: "The 3 to 11 laboratory shift always screws things up."

ER Nurse: "They sure do."

Physician: "They complain about being busy. They should spend a few days with us."

Nurse: "That would open their eyes."

Physician: "I think they are just plain lazy."

Nurse: "You are right on target."

Analysis: Here an insecure physician directs attention away from his own inadequacies with a constant stream of fault-finding remarks directed elsewhere.

The game IF IT WERE NOT FOR THEM is closely related. Here other people get blamed for anything that goes wrong or for anything not accomplished by the complaining party: "If it were not for administration…" "If it were not for that quality assurance coordinator," etc.

Games to Provoke Problems Rather Than to Solve Them

Uproar

    Medical Records Supervisor: "Well, the laboratory really caused a snafu this weekend. It will take us a month to get our records back in order."

    Laboratory Information System Coordinator: "It is too bad that your so-called specialists all have learning disorders and cannot tell us how to react to simple situations."

    Analysis: Both players avoid the difficult task of tracking down the problem and solving it. Instead they end up shouting at each other and finally walking off the scene.

How to Avoid Game Playing

The sure way to avoid initiating games ourselves is to identify within ourselves the feelings behind our behavior and "own up" to them. Authenticity is the opposite of game playing.

When you find people are trying to trap you into their games, do not accuse them of game playing, just say that you would prefer not to get into the matter any further. In other words, stay out of the game.

REFERENCES

1. Tucker RK. *Fighting it Out With Difficult People*. Dubuque, Iowa: Kendall/Hunt Publishers; 1987.

2. Watzlawick P, Weakland J, Fisch R. *Change: Principles of Problem Formation and Problem Resolution*. New York, NY: WW Norton & Co; 1974.

3. Black K. Staffing to win: an interview with Lou Holtz. *LAMA Review*. 1991;3:1.

4. Berne E. *Games People Play: The Psychology of Human Relationships*. New York, NY: Grove Press; 1964.

12.   Difficult or Just Different

No two people are exactly alike. The greater the differences in age, race, nationality, language, culture, religion, political affiliation, ethos, and personality, the greater the potential for interpersonal incompatibilities. The result is that when we deal with people who look, think, speak, and act differently, we must adjust to these dissimilarities. Because this requires special effort, and misunderstandings often ensue, we often regard these people as being difficult when they are really just different than we are.

ASSUMPTIONS, PREJUDICES, AND STEREOTYPING

Assumptions, often responsible for our perceptions and judgments, are based largely on the life scripts we develop early in life. Prejudices and stereotyping come into play all too often. For example, when we interview job applicants we may be turned off by a man with long hair or a woman with heavy makeup. We are likely to be favorably impressed by somebody who looks like us or who went to the same school. We do not like to admit that we have these feelings. Often they reside deep in our psyche. When we recognize and acknowledge these incongruities, however, we have taken a giant step toward better relationships with employees who are not really difficult people—only a little different.

THE MANY DIFFERENT DIFFERENCES

Some personality variances are perfectly compatible in certain work situations but incompatible in others. For example:

- An extroverted boss likes to have some introspective subordinates to handle jobs that require detailed attention. But, that same boss goes bananas when she has to cope with the perfectionism of an introspective colleague while working on a new project.
- Phil refers to his immaculate desk as the deck of a battleship—always ready for action. He frequently makes disparaging remarks about Alice's messy office. Phil and Alice do not get along too well, partly because of their contrasting concepts of neatness.
- Steve is chronically impatient. At a slowly paced meeting, Steve wiggles in his chair, drums his fingers on the table, and urges the supervisor to move on. At the same meeting, Ray is relaxed, enjoys the repartee, and shows it.

Before concluding that we are dealing with a difficult person, we should examine our own perceptions, assumptions, and preferences, and we should analyze those of the other person. Then we can readjust how we perceive the other person and react in a positive way to these perceptions.

Let's now start by learning more about ourselves and the people with whom we associate.

McCLELLAND'S MOTIVATIONAL NEED CLASSIFICATION

David McClelland,[1] back in the 1960s, postulated that we all have three primary motivational work needs: (1) the need to achieve; (2) the need for friends; and (3) the need for power. The intensity of these needs varies from person to person. Achievers are task-oriented; affiliators are people-oriented; and power brokers are control-oriented.

Lynn, who has a strong need for power, was delighted when she was promoted to supervisor. Now she can control what goes on around her. Lynn knows that Alex, a senior member of her staff, enjoys his professional work and does not want to be responsible for the performance of other employees. So Lynn was not surprised when Alex turned down her offer of promotion to assistant supervisor. Alex's strong motivational need is for personal task achievement. Lynn does not perceive Alex as a difficult person.

Lynn finds it more difficult to cope with the behavior of Pam, who has a strong affiliation or social need. Pam just wants to be part of the work group. She is likable, talkative, and has friends throughout the hospital. Lynn has trouble accepting Pam's long breaks, long personal phone calls, long chats in the corridor, tendency to be late for meetings, and problem with getting reports in on time. From Lynn's perspective, Pam is a difficult person. Lynn will have to adjust to Pam's marginal productivity or try to change Pam's behavior.

LEFT BRAIN/RIGHT BRAIN

Some people perceive the world through their eyes and ears (sensing). Others rely more on what springs forth from the depths of their subconscious mind (intuition).[2] The "sensors" are "left brain"–oriented while the intuitive folks are "right brain"–oriented.

The left brain people are objective, logical, and highly rational. They depend on policies, procedures, and sequential reasoning. The right brain people are subjective, innovative, and moved by gut reactions. They eschew sequential reasoning in favor of "hop-skip-and-jump" problem solving.

People who always think logically (left brain) may have difficulty getting along with intuitive (right brain) individuals whom they regard as somewhat flaky because they keep coming up with ideas that lack statistical validity. The intuitive people often complain about their rational bosses who squelch their innovative suggestions.

To determine whether you favor rationalization or innovative thinking, take the simple quiz in Table 12.1.

THE FIVE MAJOR TEMPERAMENT TYPES

Bates and Keirsey[3] found that differing temperament types can cause much interpersonal discord. The better we understand these various types, and our own, the easier it is to change our perceptions about individuals with whom we have unpleasant relationships. The following classification is based on the categories originally described by these two investigators and modified by numerous writers and seminar leaders.

1. DIRECTOR (Power Broker, Leader, Administrator, Driver)
2. PROMOTER (Salesperson, Extrovert, Troubleshooter or Troublemaker)
3. TEAM PLAYER (Loyal Soldier, Supporter, Affiliator)
4. ANALYST (Scientist, Technical Specialist, Introvert)
5. INNOVATOR (Inventor, Entrepreneur)

Instructions: To determine your predominant cognitive style, answer these five questions.

1. When you have a difficult problem, do you:
   a) Get all the facts, then figure out the best solution?
   b) Put in on the back burner—"sleep on it"?
2. When faced with change, do you:
   a) Get worried or uncomfortable?
   b) Get excited?
3. When given a new assignment, do you:
   a) Get as much information as you can about how to do it?
   b) Prefer to know only what to do, not how to do it?
4. When putting together a complicated toy, do you:
   a) Read all the directions carefully, study the diagrams, and check to see if all the parts are present?
   b) Glance at the diagrams and start putting it together?
5. When your "gut reaction" differs from the facts, do you:
   a) Almost always follow the logical course?
   b) Tend to follow your "gut reaction"?

Interpretation: If you selected mostly (a) responses, you prefer logical reasoning. If you selected mostly (b) responses, you prefer to rely on your intuition.

Table 12.1 Logical Reasoning vs Intuition.

The Director

Directors like to be in control. They are decisive, self-confident, and efficient. They work at a fast pace and are results-oriented, determined, and competitive. Their dress is formal, desks uncluttered, and office decor on the sparse side. While most of them prefer verbal communication, some are prolific senders of written messages—especially memos.

Directors are practical, organized, industrious, committed, dependable, ambitious, and bottom-line–oriented. They can see the big picture and are effective leaders. Their potential limitations are that they tend to be bureaucratic, dogmatic, stubborn, rigid, distant, critical, driving, insensitive. They are irritated by radical ideas, laziness, lateness, emotion, and ambiguity.

A potential problem with followers who possess director temperaments but who are subordinates is that they may confront and challenge their superiors—even taking over when a leader shows signs of weakness. These individuals often become informal or union leaders. On the other hand, when they are arrogant, intimidating, or self-serving, their peers may turn against them.

The key to handling directors who are subordinates is to offer them leadership roles while maintaining overall control and preventing them from misusing their authority. This authority must be defined clearly and the limits known to all individuals within its scope.

Leadership opportunities are plentiful. Let these people represent you at meetings, chair committees, and head projects or satellite activities. If they get out of control or become uncooperative, disloyal, or marginally productive, you must counsel, discipline, or remove them from leadership roles.

A common problem develops when a young outsider is brought in to head a unit in which an older subordinate director has been passed over. The new supervisor must be firm and insist on satisfactory performance from the resentful person.

The Promoter

Promoters are on the flamboyant side. Their work space is cluttered with plaques and photographs of people—especially important ones. They are spontaneous, people-oriented, emotional, dynamic, entertaining, and warm. They thrive in crises and are always in the middle of any action or confrontation. They eschew written communications.

Promoters usually are courageous, optimistic, enthusiastic, cheerful, socially skilled, confident, persuasive, and energetic. They can be risk-takers and motivators. Some are inspirational, even charismatic.

On the negative side, promoters may be pushy, intimidating, impulsive, manipulative, and careless. They may lack continuity, forget promises, and take liberties with figures and facts. Promoters are irritated by lack of enthusiasm, waiting, indecision, paperwork, monotonous tasks, and being told how they must do things.

When promoters are clients or superiors, be effervescent and enthusiastic. Relate stories and do not hurry discussion. Be friendly and informal. Ask about their family. Use open-ended questions. Do not press for decisions until socializing time has expired. Show flexibility and willingness to compromise.

When promoters are subordinates, minimize assignments that require details, paperwork, or monotonous tasks. Do not force them to work alone. Use them in public relations or sales. They are superb achievers in annual fund drives. Put them in charge of planning social events or orientation programs. Let them represent you at meetings where persuasion rather than knowledge of details is required. They are great troubleshooters.

Give them leeway in how things are to be done. But, although you permit a loose rein, keep your eyes on these eager beavers. They can get you in trouble. They can be troublemakers as well as troubleshooters—do not let them promise things that your department cannot deliver.

The Team Player

Team players seek conformity in appearance and actions. They are people-oriented. Pictures of family members adorn their desks or work areas.

These friendly folks are super-sociable and loyal. Their performance is variable, and they need closer supervision and occasional prods. They are away from their work areas a lot—in transit or at the workstations of fellow workers.

Team players are good communicators. Neurolinguistically speaking, they make maximum use of all communication modalities. They listen well, talk often, send and receive powerful visual messages, and do a lot of touching. They are the principal transmitters in the organizational grapevine.

Patience and understanding are featured by team players, who care a great deal about the feelings of others. They avoid conflict, make peace, and promote harmony. They talk a lot about teamwork and compatibility. They find it hard to say "no." They make great caregivers!

Team players work well in groups. You hear a lot of talking, kidding, and laughing in these groups. These teams are not always highly productive unless there is also a good leader. Team players are caring, friendly, helpful, accessible, trusting, loyal, great listeners, and peacemakers. In addition to great teamwork, they have a low turnover rate.

Conversely, team players tend to be indecisive, hesitant, vulnerable, impractical, and subjective. Their productivity varies, and they have difficulty managing time. They often overpromise or overcommit. Team players are irritated by conflict or dissension, being ignored, insincerity, close supervision, and rigid rules.

These employees take up more of your time. They require a tighter rein, but without harassment. Establish short-term goals that include deadlines and productivity levels.

They must have the opportunity to socialize and to interact with peers. Like promoters, they are very helpful in making new employees feel welcome, and they function well as committee members. Consider these attributes when selecting assignments that require teamwork and personality compatibilities.

Recognize the value of their friendliness and caring attitudes—and tell them. Soften criticism—their feelings are easily hurt. Do not put them in high-conflict arenas. Discuss feelings and opinions rather than debating facts and logic.

Do not pressure them for immediate decisions or take advantage of their tendency to give in without expressing how they really feel about things.

Show loyalty to them individually and as a group. Protect them against hostile outsiders. Defend them against those who take advantage of their vulnerability.

The Analyst

Analysts are productive hard workers who always score well on performance appraisals and are often promoted. They are task-oriented, reserved, formal, and conservative. Their work area is tidy and organized. Decorations are in the form of charts, graphs, or licenses. They are prompt, exacting, practical, and reliable. They prefer written communication.

Analysts often prefer to work alone. This can be a problem because teamwork is becoming increasingly important in health care institutions.

When these workers are workaholics—and they often are—they are prone to burnout. When they are perfectionists, they can be a pain—appearing aloof, hypercritical, condescending, and unpopular with their associates.

When analysts become supervisors, they are often reluctant to give up their former tasks and try to perform both as a doer and a manager. Little wonder that so many become frustrated and overstressed.

Their strong features are that they are accurate, factual, practical, meticulous, serious, industrious, thorough, consistent, and persistent.

Their limitations are manifested when they are aloof, impatient, withdrawn, critical, sullen, and negative. Their perfectionism can delay results. They are often poor delegators and can be reluctant to take risks or to accept change. Analysts are irritated by subjectivity, poor logic, idle chatter, and loss of privacy.

The Innovator

Innovators live in a chronic state of restlessness. They believe that there is always a better way of doing things. They are individualistic employees who ignore bureaucratic procedures, shun set schedules, and buck anything that they regard as obstacles to change. They like challenges with the same intensity as they dislike obstacles to change.

Innovators are optimistic risk-takers who rarely talk about failure. They often appear to be preoccupied and have the ability to turn on both their rational and intuitive thought processes. They have insatiable curiosity and sensitivity to problems.

The generation of new ideas is their strong suit. They are also enthusiastic, optimistic, and willing to take risks. They are both persistent and tolerant of ambiguity and isolation.

Innovators may annoy superiors because of their nontraditional approaches and their persistence. They are not the best team members, and they may appear uncooperative. Innovators are irritated by what they perceive as restrictive leadership. They are turned off by routines, rules, and rigid schedules.

Identify these individuals whose predominant temperament is that of creativity. Still better, seek out the latent innovativeness of all of your employees—we all have some. Be alert for statements that begin with "Why don't we...?" "What if...?" or "I wish someone would...." These are all ideas waiting to be born. Do not destroy the newborn idea by ridiculing the suggestions. If you do, you will not get any more.

Use the PIC response to all ideas:

P = Positive. If you find an idea worthwhile, say so: "Great idea—let's try it." "What can I do to help?"

I = Interesting. If you want to hear more, say, "That sounds interesting, tell me more."

C = Concern. If you cannot find anything of value in the idea, say that you have some concerns and express them. Avoid killing the suggestion directly with a negative comment such as, "The problem with that is...."

To bring out creativity in others you must overcome your ideonarcissism. Ideonarcissism is the egotism of thinking that your ideas are always unique, and because of your vast experience, your solutions must be the best ones.

The creative urge is stimulated by challenge and inhibited by routines. The innovators thrive on problems that only they can solve, so make use of that talent. Give them a loose rein to pursue and develop new ideas. Tolerate some daydreaming. They need this to fire up their creativity engine or to retrieve some information stuck in the depths of their subconscious minds.

If necessary, try to release them from monotonous tasks and rigid schedules. Allow them some discretionary time for nondirected research. The people who are already spending their personal time so engaged on weekends are the most deserving.

Tolerate failures and regard them as learning experiences. Support and protect them. Employees and managers may harass these people because they are "different."

Reward them appropriately for their good ideas. Shower them with recognition. Encourage them to publish their works. Permit them to attend scientific meetings where they can exchange ideas with other creative people.

WHAT IS YOUR PRIMARY TEMPERAMENT?

To find your predominant temperament, take the quiz in Table 12.2. After you have done this for your own temperament, determine that of the person with whom you are having the most difficulty. You will probably find that you fit into different groups.

Instructions: Underline the terms in each column that describe you. Then, add up the number of underlined items in each column.

Like people	Like action	Like plans	Like tasks	Like change
Dislike memos	Dislike memos	Prefer memos	Prefer memos	Intuitive
Caring	Risk taker	Practical	Exacting	Sense of humor
Supportive	Competitive	Direct	Thorough	Creative
Optimistic	Optimistic	Conservative	Intellectual	Spontaneous
Enthusiastic	Enthusiastic	Factual	Factual	Artistic
Trusting	Open	Traditional	Reserved	Plays hunches
Sensitive	Direct	Dependable	Practical	Innovative
Talkative	Talkative	Organized	Organized	Risk taker
Emotional	Emotional	Unemotional	Unemotional	Optimistic
Peacemaker	Outgoing	Economical	Risk avoider	Independent
Loyal	Like change	Hate stress	Hate risk	Skeptical
Popular	Restless	Determined	Perfectionist	Curious
Sociable	Courageous	Industrious	Meticulous	Impatient
Soft hearted	Persuasive	Ambitious	Objective	Preoccupied
Agreeable	Confident	Cautious	Cautious	Like challenge
Patient	Flamboyant	Prepared	Analytical	Many ideas
Cooperative	Dynamic	Logical	Logical	Enthusiastic
Personable	Impulsive	Responsible	Persistent	Dislike routine
Relaxed	Excitable	Impatient	Impatient	Nontraditional

Interpretation: Your temperament type is indicated by the column that contains the most underlined characteristics.

Column 1: Team Player

Column 2: Promoter

Column 3: Director

Column 4: Analyst

Column 5: Innovator

Table 12.2 Determining Your Primary Temperament Type

It is unlikely that either of you want or can change these characteristics, but a better understanding of how you are different will help you to cope with the other person's behavior. For example, if you are a DIRECTOR, you may be annoyed by PROMOTERS or TEAM PLAYERS who show up late for meetings, take long breaks, and seem to waste time socializing. On the other hand, PROMOTERS and TEAM PLAYERS cannot understand why you get so upset when they are a little late or they receive frequent personal telephone calls.

Once we recognize the primary motivational needs of an employee, we can usually take steps to satisfy those needs. This results in taking advantage of employees' strengths. For example:

- John, the PROMOTER, is responsible for explaining the new benefits package at a staff meeting. He also is in charge of the departmental orientation program and does a great job introducing new hires to staffers.
- Beatrice, a DIRECTOR, chairs several departmental committees and represents the radiology service at the hospital safety committee meetings.
- Bob, a TEAM PLAYER, organizes the departmental social events and serves on several committees in a nonleadership role.
- Jean, a ANALYST, gets a lion's share of the more difficult technical or professional assignments.
- Mike, an INNOVATOR, is working out the kinks of several new procedures.

The conclusion to be drawn from this material is that the more ways we are dissimilar to another person, the greater is the potential for conflict, and the greater effort we must make to render these variances irrelevant. The more we understand our own perceptions and temperaments, as well as those of others, the easier it is to fine-tune the interpersonal skills needed to get along with people at work and outside of work. When we feel uncomfortable around certain people, we should not label them as difficult until we are certain that it is not just a case of those people being a little different.

REFERENCES

1. McClelland DC. *The Achieving Society*. Princeton, NJ: Van Nostrand Co; 1961.
2. Myers IB, McCaulley MH. A Guide to the Development and Use of the Myer-Briggs Type Indicator. Palo Alto, Calif: Consulting Psychologists Press Inc; 1985.
3. Bates M, Keirsey DW. *Please Understand Me*. Upland, Calif: Gnosology Books Ltd; 1984.

13. The High-Tech Professional

Before we leave the subject of people who may be perceived as difficult only because they are different and sometimes must be handled differently, we must discuss the high-tech professional (HTP). The term "high-tech" differentiates these special people from other professionals such as nurses and administrators. The HTPs include physicians, laboratory scientists, researchers, and technical experts such as computer specialists. This chapter is dedicated to the managers who are serving in hospitals and hospital laboratories for the first time and find that they must deal with people who are not like themselves or the people they worked with elsewhere.

Do HTPs merit special attention? Broadwell and House[1] seem to think so, since they have written an entire book about these individuals.

Once upon a time, most hospital managers were promoted from within—from the technical or professional ranks of the institution—and they often accepted leadership roles reluctantly. For example, laboratory technologists became laboratory supervisors and laboratory supervisors became chief medical technologists. These individuals often lacked supervisory training, but nevertheless they got the job done, often with outstanding success.

The past decade, however, has seen an influx of managers who have no medical or hospital background. Most are graduates of business schools or are transplants from commercial enterprises.

Enter the MBAs, and trouble brewed. These "outsiders" are often still regarded with suspicion by medical and nursing personnel. The HTPs for the first time

111

reported to individuals who were not familiar with the HTPs' work or attitude. The HTPs also watched the erosion of their responsibility, autonomy, self-image, and status. For example, a middle-aged physician who headed a clinical laboratory now found himself sharing a leadership role with a young laboratory manager and reporting to a young MBA vice president of medical affairs instead of directly to the CEO as he had in the past.

Business school graduates are sometimes surprised and frustrated by these individualistic, intelligent HTPs who often ignore bureaucratic procedures, shun set schedules, and resist attempts to make them more efficient. Because of these characteristics, Geber[2] refers to the HTPs as "wild ducks." Clashes due to differences in values, autonomy, status, and remuneration were inevitable. Undercurrents of disagreement, animosity, and distrust grew.

One major difference between hospitals and other businesses is the presence in hospitals of the medical staff. The medical staff has its own officers, its own rules and regulations (the bylaws), and its own disciplinary measures. On top of all that, the attending physicians are major customers and expect to be treated as such. You will meet some of the not-so-nice ones in subsequent chapters.

WHY ARE HTPs DIFFERENT?

High-tech professionals are different for several reasons. In the first place, individuals whose interests are in medicine, microbiology, chemistry, histology, pharmacy, or some other art or science, and who receive intensive training in the arts or sciences, march to a different drummer than do individuals whose education focuses on accounting, business principles, management, marketing, and economics.

A difference also exists in the nature of the tasks performed by these two groups. The laboratorian, for example, deals with scientific tasks and strives to achieve perfection—zero defects. The business person is more interested in customer satisfaction and return on investment.

Fortunately, many health care professionals now receive training in both the healing arts and business administration. In the laboratory, MD-MBA degrees are becoming as commonplace as MD-PhDs. Many medical technologists are acquiring business degrees. This kind of cross-training helps to eliminate attitudinal incompatibilities.

CHARACTERISTICS OF HTPs

At the risk of unwarranted stereotyping, we would like to describe certain characteristics that HTPs exhibit to a greater degree than do other groups.

For example, HTPs often exhibit greater loyal to their profession than to their superiors. While it is important for them to be respected by their professional peers, they often have only marginal interest in winning the approval of administrators. They are highly focused on their own specialty, and they strive for technical excellence. Most are extremely competent and take great pride in their accomplishments. They often know more than their supervisors about specific areas of expertise.

HTPs are often impatient, especially with any organizational requirement that interferes with their work. This impatience is sometimes interpreted as lack of cooperation. They may be curt with people who lack their knowledge or education, and they tend not to mix with nontechnical people, often being conspicuous by their absence at staff social affairs.[1]

Some HTPs have big egos, and a few are difficult to control because they develop a prima donna complex. Confident of their job skills or knowledge, they feel secure and irreplaceable. They may become abrasive to others, even to customers. Such attitudes and behavior can have a devastating effect on customer service and departmental morale.[3] On the other hand, some HTPs suffer from low self-esteem and complain bitterly about lack of recognition or appreciation.

A minority of these people aspire to join the managerial ranks. When they are promoted to supervisory posts, many are unhappy in that role and wish that they could go back to doing "professional" work. This is also seen in universities where many professors happily return to teaching after a stint as dean or department chief.

Mandatory management training may strike HTPs as a waste of time, and they may react to it by ignoring the trainers or making fun of them. They may actually enjoy seeing management discomforted. They hate administrative paperwork and have little tolerance for those who do it. They often regard colleagues who move into administrative roles as less competent professionals.

The many subsets of this group are defined by their varying degrees of interest in teaching, participating in professional societies, publishing, and serving on committees. Some are highly creative, others are not. Some are good team players, but most are task-directed rather than people-oriented.

Some members of this group have problems integrating into the formal and informal structure of organizations. They eschew conformity and repeatedly proclaim their independence. They want and expect technical freedom and dislike routine work and schedules.

They may be unconventional in habits and appearance, often violating or bending rules. While they may come in late or leave early, they usually spend long hours on the job and are frequently found in their work areas on weekends and holidays. They are not clock watchers.

HTPs want to practice elegant procedures, while management pressures them for faster results. They seek autonomy of the conditions, pace, and content of their work, while management wants to keep them on course.[4]

Because HTPs are often more loyal to their profession than to their employer, their lay managers regard them with suspicion. The latter often perceive HTPs as politically naive, petulant, aloof, indifferent, and even disloyal. It is hard for these managers to understand why these people have trouble supporting a policy that the manager sees as good for the organization.[4]

HOW TO HANDLE HTPs

Job Applicants

Try to identify prima donnas and other potential problem people during the selection process. Avoid the professionals who are most likely to have role conflicts. Ask applicants to describe their work style and to relate examples of their ability to work as part of a team. Question them about their goals and aspirations, and then match these with those of your organization. Ask their references how the applicants got along with others.[3] Be frank about the opportunities in your department for advancement. Do you have a clinical ladder or are promotions only into administration? Is it publish or perish?[4]

Orientation

During the orientation phase, be very explicit as to the responsibilities involved and the degrees of autonomy permitted. Emphasize the importance of customer service and budget restrictions. If the new hires find that they dislike the restrictions imposed on them, or they yearn for the academic atmosphere they left behind, it is much better for all parties for them to discover this during their probationary period.

Leadership Style

Managers are caught between the demands of hospital administrators and the demands for autonomy and support by those they supervise.[1] Health care managers deal with a great variety of workers, from those who are mentally challenged to people with advanced educational degrees; those who require constant direction to others who thrive and are most productive when working autonomously. This calls for a flexible or situational leadership style. Leaders must tailor their style to that most appropriate for each subordinate and each work situation. A delegative or consultative leadership style is best when dealing with experienced professionals. Supervisory control is minimal and group leaders function as coordinators and facilitators. They remove obstacles, bend rules, cut red tape, remove distractions, and run interference. They permit flexible schedules when feasible. They empower, provide autonomy, present challenges, and ensure the availability of the necessary resources.

A challenging job is one in which HTPs find ways to use their professional skills and the new ones they learn. "The nemesis of challenge is underutilization of skills. Denied the opportunity to grow in the job, [the HTP] becomes bored, apathetic, and subject to deviance, burnout, or alienation."[4]

A "leave-alone" style is not always appropriate. If a neophyte is turned loose without adequate supervision, he may perform poorly and then get zapped by superiors. This ends in that employee's demoralization and his fear of taking on any additional risks. Even in the case of experienced professionals, their managers must determine the "what" while leaving the "how" up to the HTP.

Involve them more in decision making, problem solving, and formulating policies and guidelines. Invite and respect their opinions and suggestions. Demonstrate trust and confidence in their competency.

Horizontal Leadership

Health care supervisors are now faced with an additional challenge and one that involves the HTPs—the need to obtain the cooperation of people over whom they have no authority. The current paradigm shift playing out in hospitals features cross-functional teams, especially in the implementation of quality improvement programs and cost-reduction measures. New committees, focus groups, quality circles, and brainstorming sessions all call for a degree of coordination and cooperation never before required. Horizontal leadership is becoming as important as supervision that follows traditional vertical channels.

Supervisors must become effective negotiators and demonstrate superior persuasiveness. To achieve this, they must earn the respect of all the employees with whom they interact, especially the HTPs.

Recognition and Rewards

Provide performance feedback in objective terms related to task performance rather than to personality or attitude. Conversely, never tolerate poor customer service or abuse of coworkers.

Fight for merit rewards for the individuals and work teams who provide valuable service but whose records are slightly tarnished by minor compatibility problems or slight lack of conformity. Avoid rewarding marginal performers. This precipitates anger and resentment among the HTPs.[5]

Communication

Learn the fundamentals and terminology of their specialty. Provide opportunities for them to share their professional knowledge by attending professional meetings or giving lectures or workshops. Broadcast congratulatory news such as results of special projects, research developments, and individual achievements.[5]

Educational and Training Opportunities

Encourage the HTPs' continuing education but do not force them into supervisory training against their wishes. These people thrive on attending technical and professional meetings. Approve as many as you can—they deserve higher priorities than many health care employers give them. Provide opportunities for them to use the skills they learn. Make appropriate reference books and periodicals available.

If these employees have compatibility problems, encourage them to attend remedial seminars on interpersonal relationships. Be diplomatic but persistent when you suggest these. A good time is at annual performance reviews. At staff meetings, emphasize the importance of teamwork and explain that lack of cooperation destroys teams. Reinforce any attempt the employee makes at being more sociable or accommodating.

Insist on acceptable performance and do not reward poor behavior. Counsel on the necessity for HTPs to pitch in and help when necessary. Use peer pressure to reinforce group norms. Do not bend the rules too far for them.[3]

To prevent the prima donna complex, use cross-training so that other employees can substitute for the superstar, should that become necessary. A good time to initiate this is before the prima donna takes his next vacation.

The Nonconformist

The nonconformist requires special handling, which is not always easy. This is complicated when the nonconformist possesses expertise that is scarce and essential. You know this, and so does the nonconformist. Weiss[6] recommends asking yourself these three key questions:

1. Does their upbeat lifestyle affect work results?
2. Do they disrupt the efforts of other employees?
3. If you accept them as they are, will that arouse resentment in other employees who perceive the nonconformist as receiving favored treatment?

If your answers indicate that employee's idiosyncrasies are not really detrimental to performance or team effort, it is probably best for you to adjust to the situation. Surprisingly, once you do that, you will usually find that there was not such a big problem after all.[6]

Let them know that you regard them as valuable members of the work unit. Tolerate their impatience and complaints. Do not accuse them of being stubborn or unreasonable. Bend the rules a bit—but not too far.[7] Make them accountable for results but release them from rigid schedules. Ask them for their advice before setting new goals.

REFERENCES

1. Broadwell MM, House RS. *Supervising Technical and Professional People*. New York, NY: John Wiley & Sons; 1986.

2. Geber B. How to manage wild ducks. *Training*. 1990;27:5.

3. Osborne JE. Supervising superstars: the talent and temperament conflict. *Supervis Manage*. 1991;36:4-5.

4. Raelin J, Sholl CK, Leonard D. Why professionals turn sour and what to do. *Personnel*. 1985;2:8-41.

5. Lea D, Brostrom R. Managing the high-tech professional. *Personnel*. 1988;65:12-22.

6. Weiss WH. *The Supervisor's Problem Solver*. New York, NY: AMACOM; 1982.

7. Glassman E. Understanding and supervising low conformers. *Supervis Manage*. 1990;35:11.

14. Difficult People at Meetings

Meetings are the best place to practice your people-coping skills, especially when turf, dollars, or personnel changes are being discussed. At a single meeting you can come up against all sorts of annoying characters. If you are the moderator, it is your responsibility to keep them all in check.

HOW TO RUN AN EFFICIENT MEETING

The more efficiently a meeting is conducted, the fewer will be the problems encountered. When meetings drag on without much being accomplished, when aggressive members dominate discussions, when the room is uncomfortable, when the coffee fails to materialize, and when arguments are permitted to escalate, the participants get irritable, impatient, and testy. Even the usually mild-mannered folks get their dander up.

Meeting Preparations Are Important

The first step in preparing for a meeting is to determine who should attend. Avoid having too many people—the fewer the merrier. Often, problem participants are people who need not or should not be present and who become disrupters. The group should collectively have the knowledge and experience needed. Include people who have the power to make decisions, people who will be responsible for implementing those decisions, and people who represent groups that are affected by the decisions.

Since power disparity inhibits frank discussions, it should be minimized. This is the responsibility of the chair. If the chair is the power broker, the meeting is doomed. Although you do not want negativists present, every group meeting should have a "devil's advocate" who asks penetrating questions but who, unlike negativists, does not seek to derail the negotiations.

To reduce the number of attendees at a regularly scheduled meeting, encourage certain members to skip that particular meeting, but without offending them. Most members will appreciate your consideration of their time. For example: "Alice, this next meeting has nothing that pertains directly to your area of responsibility or expertise. We will deal only with maintenance contracts. You are welcome to attend, but if you choose not to come, we will understand."

If you do not need your boss's presence, and she tends to dominate meetings, find a diplomatic way to discourage her presence. For example: "Tammy, I know you are very busy. You may want to skip this next session. Here is the agenda. Is there anything that you would like me to express on your behalf?"

If you seek support for a favorite project, ask yourself who will support it, who will oppose it, and who is likely to be undecided. You may want to discuss your proposal with some of these people prior to the meeting. If you anticipate problems with a particular person, talk this over with some of the other members before the meeting and solicit their support. For example: "Eileen, I am afraid that Lewis will try to stonewall our attempt to get the figures on the new wellness program. You have a way of getting Lewis to cooperate. Would you be willing to pressure him to come up with those statistics?"

Have any proposal you plan to make written down, preferably in the form of a motion, especially if it is a complicated one. State your recommendations with specific terminology in terms of action and objectivity. No confusion should exist as to what results are to be achieved. Instead of saying, "Try to improve cooperation with materials management," state, "Hold a joint meeting with materials management twice a year."

On the agenda, indicate the amount of time allocated for each item. Send out the agenda early enough for the members to arrange their schedules. Before you select a definite date and time, call key members to ensure their availability. Make certain that the visual aids and necessary amenities will be available. A committee wandering around the halls looking for a free room deserves a new program chair or facilitator.

It is Starting Time!

Start on time, even when only a few people are present. If this is a regularly scheduled event, members will come earlier once they realize that the meetings always begin as scheduled. Conversely, when meetings start late, members will arrive later and later. Stand at the door and greet people as they arrive. Make any necessary introductions.

Seating Arrangements Are Important

To establish an egalitarian atmosphere, seat people in a circle or chevron arrangement; avoid classroom seating. Encourage antagonists to sit side by side rather than across from each other. If two people always sit at the end of a long table and carry on private conversations, seat them near you or put a serious attentive person between them.

Discuss less important items first, saving the biggies for when everyone is present and people have not yet started to drift off.

Sound enthusiastic and say something to emphasize the importance of the meeting. Avoid the verb "discuss," which suggests talk but no action. Use an action statement. For example: "Before we leave this room, we must come up with a recommendation for cutting our capital equipment budget by 25%."

Use Powerful Body Language

Sit erect. To project interest, lean slightly forward toward a speaker and make eye contact. Take up space by putting some of your materials, such as a notebook or folder, on the table. Occasionally rest your forearm on the edge of the table. Do not put your hands on your lap or fold your arms across your chest.

Stand up and erect when you make a proposal or offer a rebuttal, unless this is a very small group.

Watch your facial expression when listening to others. If you are the moderator, your facial expression should not reveal approval or disapproval—only polite interest. On the other hand, if you are not the chair, do show how you feel by smiles, frowns, and nods.

Maintain Control by Facilitating, Not Dominating

Use the "around-the-table" approach to draw everyone out. Ask open-ended, nonthreatening questions (eg, "How do you think the nursing service will react to that?").

Summarize progress periodically, preferably by using a flip chart or chalkboard. Do not jump to a vote too soon. Instead, strive for a consensus or an agreement by all attendees that they can live with the decision even though it is not the first choice of all. Reinforce desired behavior (eg, "Marilyn, thank you for speaking so candidly. That took courage"). Call for a break or a stretch when things stall. Then continue if the members seem to be up to it. If interest is flagging or the participants look beat, it is best to conclude the meeting, unless items are on the agenda that must be addressed at that time.

Some Important Don'ts

- Dominate discussions.
- Take sides or tell participants that they are wrong.
- Intimidate, ridicule, kid, or be sarcastic.
- Make sotto voce comments to the person sitting next to you.
- Instruct or lecture.
- Permit emotional arguments to develop. When disagreements grow tense, get back to the agenda or call a break.
- Show impatience by tapping your fingers or pen on the table, shuffling papers, glancing at your watch, or cutting off people in the middle of their sentences.
- Try to be a comedian—a little humor is appropriate, but not at someone else's expense.
- Show resentment over a remark or take criticism personally.
- Make dogmatic statements—they irritate people and start arguments.
- Get into long debates—state your case and let others take up the discussion.
- Permit the meeting to run over the time allowed.

THE DIFFICULT PARTICIPANTS

No matter how well a meeting is planned and executed, there will always be difficult participants who will make the proceedings interesting.

The Habitually Late Arrivers

Do not fill late participants in on what has transpired, unless they are key members. Tardiness needs to be modified by negative reinforcement. If they insist on getting a summary, give it hurriedly with an overtone of annoyance or ask the person seated next to them to do so.

The Bosses Who Like to Take Over

Nip the problem of a dominating boss in the bud by disinviting her. If the boss still plans to attend, clue her in as to what you perceive her contribution to be. At the meeting give a signal when it is a good time for the boss to leave. For example:

> (before meeting): "Grace, if you attend our meeting, I would appreciate your support for the recognition program we talked about last week."
> (at the meeting): "Thanks, Dr. Allison, for those succinct remarks. It was good of you to meet with us. Please feel free to stay for the rest of the meeting, but I know that you have a very busy schedule."

Quick[1] contends that if your boss still takes over your meetings, it probably means that she does not think you are doing a very good job as moderator.

The Intimidators

Intimidation is a common method for forcing opinions onto others. The intimidator often has worthwhile suggestions but wants to ram ideas through without any discussion. Intimidation is an emotional process that requires fear to be effective. The tactics can be to appear angry, to ridicule, or to assume a superior attitude.

Do not get into a battle by immediately countering the intimidator's statements. If you do that, you will appear to be obstructive or you will find yourself in a battle royal. Conversely, if you remain silent, the intimidator will interpret that as acquiescence. If you do attempt a head-on confrontation, be sure that you have the group's support.

Instead of counterattacking or remaining silent, ask other members to speak up. If they do and are put down by the dominator, rush to the offended member's defense. Never permit a member to mock, ridicule, or insult another member. For example: "Larry, that reaction is uncalled for. I do not appreciate it and I am sure the others here agree. Let's keep this professional." Apologize on behalf of the group to the person who has been offended.

If no other member takes on an intimidator, it is up to you to do so. As you respond, direct your remarks to the group rather than solely to the intimidator. Ask the members specific questions about the proposal. If the intimidator objects and wants a vote, reply that you want more discussion. For example: "Larry, I do not think we are ready to vote on that. In fact, I would prefer that we seek a consensus rather than a majority vote," or, "Larry, I am getting a bit upset about how you keep demanding that we take a vote."

The Know-it-alls

These self-appointed experts are condescending, pompous, and boring to everyone but themselves. They try to make everyone else feel like idiots. Do not argue with these people. If you must respond, make certain that your statements are factual and that you can provide documented facts. When the know-it-all starts pontificating, ask other members to comment.

The Motor Mouths

Some people seem enthralled by their own voices. They ramble on interminably, divert the discussion with anecdotes, and quibble over minutia.

Break off eye contact when you want these folks to stop talking. When they pause for a breath, ask them to summarize or request that they put their comments in the form of motions. If they fail to summarize, paraphrase what you have heard or ask for clarification. Then get others into the discourse. For example: "What I hear you saying, Suzanne, is.... Do I have that right?" "You have lost me, Suzanne, please explain what you mean."

If they go off on a tangent, issue a relevance challenge. For example: "Suzanne, I am confused. What you are saying does not seem to pertain to the suggestion Bob made. Am I wrong about that?" "Suzanne, that is interesting, but we are getting away from our topic."

When all else fails, plead time limitations. For example: "It is 5 minutes to 5:00, Suzanne. I would like to go around the table and get every person's thoughts on what you just said before we adjourn."

The Arguers

Two people are disputing each other's views, and the argument is going nowhere. They are starting to repeat, talking louder, interrupting each other, and getting red in the face.

Before things get out of hand, stop one of the pair and ask the other one to summarize the opponent's viewpoint. The first person will usually correctly point out that the second person's interpretation is all wrong. Reverse the process and continue until both sides agree as to what each is saying. This forces the opponents to move from personalities to topics. You have served as mediator and harmonizer. Now get the other people into the act. For example: "Well, we have an interesting difference of opinion here, and both Alice and John have presented powerful arguments for us to consider. What do you think about this, Fred?"

The Silent Ones

Because a member is silent does not mean that she has nothing important to offer. It is usually a question of assertiveness. These people are afraid that what they say will sound stupid. Their position on the pecking scale, the number of letters after their name, the length of their experience in the organization, and how their previous verbal offerings were received all impact their willingness to speak up.

Prepare "the clam" by discussing the topic with her before the meeting and telling her that you value her opinion and would like her to express it. At the meeting, say something like, "Donna, would you please repeat what you told me the other day?"

Such preparations are not always possible. Other strategies include: seating a silent member between two friendly and talkative members; drawing her out by asking simple, nonthreatening questions for starters; or making eye contact with her when putting a question to the group. The last tactic cannot be used repeatedly because reluctant responders learn to stare at the ground to prevent eye contact—a defensive response learned quickly by all students who do not want to be called on in class.

Encourage reticent participants by taking their contributions seriously and acknowledging them. For example: "That was a well thought-out opinion, Ralph. I am relieved to know that things are not as desperate as I was led to believe. Do any of you have questions for Ralph—he is obviously well informed on this topic?"

The Private Conversers

People carry on private conversations for a number of reasons. They may want to express opinions but are too timid to speak up, are bored, have urgent personal matters to relate, or are just discourteous.

If you suspect timidity, say something like, "Dana, you seem to have something to share. Please share it with all of us." Be less gentle with the other distractors. If you are talking, stop and stare at them, direct a question at one of them, or ask for their opinions.

The Hecklers and Comics

A little humor is healthy, but some participants are more interested in getting laughs than in getting results. If encouraged by laughter and smiles, they may expand their act and derail a meeting. The remedy is to show a brief, cool smile and say, "Okay, Maureen, we have had our little fun. Now let's get back to work." When she pokes fun at something or someone, ask the group how they feel about what the heckler just said.

The Hidden Agenda Holders

Suspect a hidden agenda when participants spend a lot of time bickering, seem to be reinforcing each others comments too vigorously, or one person continues to pursue a subject that is not on the agenda.[1] Their unspoken, selfish message is "I want something" or "What is in it for me?" Often this is readily apparent to the group. For example, when Ruth insists that the next meeting be held at the Hillside Restaurant, everyone knows that Ruth's choice is influenced by the fact that her uncle owns that restaurant.

If you suspect a hidden agenda, but it does not seem to impede the progress of the meeting or hurt someone's feelings, you can safely ignore it. But if it becomes obstructive, you must take action. Sometimes you can simply switch the discussion to another topic. Getting other members involved in the dialogue usually will eliminate the problem. Asking pointed questions like, "How will that benefit our patients?" may expose their selfish purposes.

The Negativists

These "wet blankets" are always the first to point out why something will not work. Their favorite statements include: "That would never work here," "We tried that before, and it was a disaster," or "Management would never go for that." They give in seldom and then only grudgingly. In chapter 21 we will explore these difficult people in greater depth.

The Destroyers

Some participants become emotionally involved. They play psychological games and attract attention by criticizing members or taking offense at innocent remarks. They may say "I resent that and I want an apology," or "If you approve that ridiculous motion, I am going to walk out of here."

Ignore these outbursts. Act as though you did not hear their threats or accusations. Do not argue or lose your temper. If ignoring them does not work, and they continue to disrupt the meeting, you must turn on the assertive strategies we describe in chapter 24 for dealing with hostile people. If they get up and walk out, let them.

REFERENCE

1. Quick TL. *Managing People at Work: Desk Guide*. New York, NY: Executive Enterprises Publications, Inc; 1983.

15.   Difficult Patients

Patients have good reasons for being difficult. People give up a lot of control over their lives when they are in the hospital. This control is transferred to providers, most of whom are total strangers. The loss of control, combined with separation from family, concern about medical outcome, fear of the future, financial concern, and discomfort or pain, produces great stress.

THE SPECIAL ROLE OF PHLEBOTOMISTS

With the exception of phlebotomists and receptionists, few laboratorians have much patient contact, which is sometimes the reason laboratory people prefer their line of work. Phlebotomists, however, do spend most of their days with patients. The role of a blood collector is not an easy one. The visits of most caregivers are pleasant ones for the patients. Nurses and physicians bring relief of pain, back rubs, trays of food, and sometimes new babies. The visits of blood collectors, on the other hand, are about as popular as those of the orderly who administers enemas—they bring pain.

Phlebotomists must be selected for their patience and caring attitude as well as for their skill with the needles. Their orientation program includes not only interactive skill training but also advice on how to (and especially how not to) answer the queries of patients, such as, "What are you going to do with that blood?" "Why are you sticking me again today?" "What will those tests show?" "Do I have cancer?" "Why doesn't my doctor visit me more often?" "Why are the nurses so grumpy?" "Do you enjoy hurting people?" "Are you the reason I get cold breakfasts?"

Supervisors who harp on the need for quick delivery of blood specimens to the laboratory make it difficult for blood collectors to show the courtesies and pleasantries that patients deserve—a matter of guest relations, again, if you like.

FIRST IMPRESSIONS ARE THE STRONGEST

Nurses commonly classify patients as "good" or "bad" within the first 24 hours of admission.[1] If the patient has had a previous unpleasant experience in a hospital, especially the same hospital, the environment is negatively charged at the time of admission. Nursing personnel frequently sense this negativism. When this impression is reinforced by the patient's lack of cooperation, the diagnosis is confirmed in the nurse's mind—a "bad" patient. Conversely, when a patient has had a good experience with a hospital, he will have a more positive interaction with his caretakers—a "good" patient.

HOW PATIENTS FEEL AND ACT

Patients may experience anger, sadness, worry, or many other emotions. Their selection of words provides clues as to which feeling predominates: "I am upset" (anger); "Nobody seems to care about me" (sadness); or "Why do you need all that blood?" (worry). When anger is self-directed, you hear, "I should have..." or "If only I had...."[2]

These emotions are expressed in many different ways. Patients may become emotionally unglued, hostile, overly dependent, impatient, unappreciative, manipulative, or nonconforming.[2] They are often verbally abusive, sometimes physically threatening. More often they demand special attention or complain constantly. They may refuse diagnostic or therapeutic procedures, even when they know that the refusals may be detrimental to their recovery.

HOSPITAL PATIENTS ARE NOT THE SAME AS HOTEL GUESTS

"Guest relations" has become a health care buzzword, and many CEOs of hospitals have introduced this concept into their organizational culture—sometimes to the dismay of their nursing staffs. It is one thing to provide valet parking and have smiling faces greet newly admitted patients. We applaud hospital CEOs who are streamlining admitting procedures, reducing waiting time in emergency rooms, making patients more comfortable, and treating all patients as special customers. On the other hand, to expect overworked and understaffed nursing and house staffs to treat patients and their families like visiting dignitaries is asking a bit too much. When the "guest relations" concept is publicized, it is difficult for hospital employees to meet or exceed patient expectations.

Additionally, Montgomery[3] points out that it is one thing to satisfy the demands of a hotel or restaurant patron, and quite another to accede to those of patients when such acquiescence is not in the best interest of the medical care. The issue becomes one of wants vs needs. Hotels can cater to the *wants* of their customers, whereas hospitals must make the *needs* of their patients the top priority. For example, when a guest orders a meal in the hotel restaurant, he can choose whatever he likes from the menu. At a hospital, however, a patient whose physician requires him to eat a low-salt diet cannot reach for the salt shaker. The patient's wants are secondary to his needs. Furthermore, it is the responsibility of the health care provider to determine the proper balance between these often-conflicting demands. Medical and nursing personnel often encounter patients who refuse to take their medication, who resist attempts to rehabilitate, or who demand dangerous doses of analgesics. Caregivers are not waitresses or store clerks. They must remain in control of the medical and nursing care.

THE TYPES OF DIFFICULT PATIENTS

Problem patients display a wide variety of responses and personality types. The challenge to the health care provider is to learn to identify and cope with each different difficulty.

The Complainers

Dealing with complaints is a daily challenge for most caregivers. Compassionate health care personnel actually encourage patients to voice their needs and to express their feelings about their care. That is good customer service. These caregivers worry that patients may suffer unnecessarily because they are too frightened or too passive to express their hurts. On the other hand, the kindest of care providers become exasperated when complaints are incessant and unjustified. Complaints come not only from patients or their family members, but also from the medical staff, superiors, subordinates, coworkers, and members of other departments. Failure to resolve complaints leaves the complainers dissatisfied and the providers frustrated and frazzled.

The Demanding Complainers

Demanding patients are also complainers. Instead of whining or crying, however, they adopt an aggressive style of remonstrating. Their complaints are accompanied by threats. They demand to talk to someone in authority. They hint that they may walk out or transfer to another facility. Possible legal action is mentioned. They seem to take satisfaction in provoking employees into angry retaliation or tears.

Luna[4] describes four steps in the "complaint spiral."

- **Step 1**. A nurse responds promptly and empathetically to a complaint: "My pain medication is not working."
- **Step 2**. The complaint is restated in stronger terms, often with one or two new gripes thrown in for good measure. The nurse is now less empathic but still tries to help. The patient's physician is contacted, and the medication or the dosage is changed.
- **Step 3**. The patient becomes angry and strident: "Nurse, can't anybody relieve my pain? Why doesn't my doctor see me? I want to see whoever is in charge here." At this point, the nurse questions other staff members and finds that they too are having problems with this patient.
- **Step 4**. Additional attempts to satisfy the patient fail or a new set of complaints emerges. Now, poorly concealed dislike between the patient and the nursing staff is apparent. The nurses feel that the patient is unreasonable; the patient regards the nurses as uncaring and hostile. Family members join in the chorus of protestations. Trust in the service erodes. In the worst case scenario, legal redress is sought.

The Verbal Abusers

Although verbal abuse is usually in response to what is perceived as unsatisfactory care, it may erupt at any time, often for the most trivial of reasons. The abuser may focus on a nurse's appearance or bedside technique or on some irrelevant event or situation.

Verbal abuse is now so common and so severe that it is regarded as a significant factor in the turnover of nursing personnel. Nurses claim that physicians are also frequent offenders. In one study, 78% of the nursing staff identified members of the medical staff as the major source of such maltreatment.[5]

While physicians are often on the receiving end of tongue lashings from patients or patients' families, the duration of such attacks seldom is as strident as that directed at nurses. Family members may employ the "trickledown" sequence by taking out their frustration on members of the housekeeping service or employees in other ancillary departments. For example, imagine the phlebotomist entering the room of a distraught patient who is looking for a victim on whom to vent his anger. The unsuspecting phlebotomist is greeted with a loud, "Here comes the vampire again. What do you do with all that blood, sell it?" A series of such encounters early in the day is enough to discourage even the most caring person.

The Manipulators

Since patients normally elicit sympathy, they can easily escalate their behavior into manipulative habits. When they shift into their manipulative mode, these people combine plays on sympathy with exaggerations of pain or suffering. Their plaintive appeals are very touching, and they are masters at getting what they want by these machinations.

Frequently they concoct wild and untrue stories of how they have been mistreated or ignored. Anyone who tries to cut through these myths becomes the target of the manipulator. Because their tales are plausible, these poor souls often create rifts among their care providers unless there is close teamwork and good communication.

The Treatment Refusers

Patients have the legal right to refuse diagnostic procedures or treatment. On rare occasions, they may show more sense than their care providers. For example, when lack of coordination of test ordering results in an almost endless series of venipunctures, the patient may dramatically draw attention to this unnecessary discomfort by refusing to allow a phlebotomist to take still another blood sample.

However, in most instances, refusals are not in the patient's best interest or may even be life threatening. For example, a postoperative patient who refuses to take deep breaths may develop pulmonary atelectasis.

RESPONSES TO DIFFICULT PATIENTS

Difficult patients elicit frustration, anger, and a feeling of being exploited on the part of caregivers. These emotions are often compounded by overlays of guilt. Typical responses by the caregivers are avoidance and distancing. Latent or overt hostility may ensue, thus aggravating the situation.

It is essential to understand that emotions are almost always part of the caregiver/patient relationship. When this is kept in mind, nurses and physicians are more likely to serve as advocates and supporters rather than adversaries. Adversarial relationships represent smoldering caldrons ready to boil over at a moment's notice.

The caring person remains alert for distress signals in words, facial expressions, or body language. Often during the initial interview, an observant professional will interrupt the questioning and verbalize his observation: "You seem upset. Would you like to talk about what is bothering you?"

Instead of classifying a patient as difficult, the caring provider searches for the cause of the troublesome behavior. Often one is dealing with a patient who finds it difficult to express what he needs or wants. Unexpressed need for reassurance, comfort, or relief from anxiety may be manifested as persistent complaining. A good start is to say that the patient has a problem, not that the patient is a problem.

The caregiver must rule out toxin- and drug-induced states. Acute toxic states may be due to severe infections and shock. Drugs, therapeutic and illicit, can produce a rainbow spectrum of signs and symptoms. Metabolic aberrations can produce all sorts of bizarre behavioral changes. Uncontrolled diabetes and uremia are among the most common of these. Psychotic states also must be ruled out.

Regard complaints or hostility as calls for help. Investigate each complaint. If it is valid—and even the worst complainer has some valid gripes—demonstrate willingness to respond to it.

Assertiveness, combined with a caring attitude, is the formula for dealing with the demanding or hostile patient. When alerted to the arrival of Mr. Jones, a patient with a disagreeable temperament, use a kind but firm approach. When you introduce yourself, say that you are going to provide competent service, but that you have five other sick patients to attend. Add that you know that Mr. Jones is going to be understanding. Then be specific as to what your service will be: "I will be dropping in to see you every hour, and every three hours you will receive your medication."

A Four-Step Coping Technique

The following approach to coping with difficult patients is a modification of that recommended by Hobbs.[6]

- **Step 1.** Describe and chart the patient's problem behavior objectively. Avoid subjective labels such as "belligerent and uncooperative." Instead, record, "Patient displays signs of aggression. On three occasions today he threw his food tray on the floor. Last night he struck an orderly who tried to catheterize him."
- **Step 2.** Identify a precipitating factor. Does the behavior follow a certain event or contact with a certain person? For example, Mary's complaining is noticeably worse after a visit with her husband. This observation alone may provide the solution to the

problem. The caregiver must approach such a situation with sensitivity. To jump to conclusions or to make accusations can be self-defeating. If the caregiver has a cordial relationship with the patient, he may comment on his observation and tactfully ask if there is anything the patient would like to discuss. Under other circumstances the best approach may be to tell the husband that you are concerned about the patient's reactions after visitations and the possible adverse effect these visits are having. Try to determine if the patient's behavior is the result of fear. Many times, a frightened patient craves reassurance or a lot of hand-holding, back rubs, and other physical contact.

■ **Step 3.** Reflect on ways in which you may have actually rewarded or reinforced untoward behavior. For example, John gets faster response to his bell when it is accompanied by loud bellowing.

■ **Step 4.** Develop a written care plan to cope with the patient's behavior. If necessary, consult a behavior specialist such as a mental health nurse.

Look for ways to avoid rewarding problem behavior while reinforcing desired deportment. When John starts yelling for his breakfast, serve him last. As you enter his room avoid eye contact or conversation. Put down his tray and leave. When he does not shout, serve him more quickly, establish eye contact, smile, and chat briefly.

Often it is necessary to solicit the cooperation of all your teammates, especially when dealing with a manipulator. You may also need the support and understanding of family members.

Role-play or simulation of actual incidents in which participants practice being verbally abusive to each other is recommended. This is especially helpful for groups who have not had training in assertiveness.

Keep in close touch with the attending physician and others who are involved in the patient's care.

Other Remedial Measures

"Fogging" was mentioned in the chapter on assertiveness, and it is worth describing again. Fogging is agreeing with part of abusive statements. For example:

Patient: "Don't you believe in relieving pain? I think you enjoy seeing someone suffer."
Nurse: "Some people do think we are immune to pain and suffering. Your medication will be right on schedule, Mrs. Smith."

"Self-disclosure" helps to relieve the stress caused by unreasonable patients. Self-disclosure is revealing how you feel about an unpleasant situation (eg, "When you shout at me, I get upset. Please stop!").

Avoidance or distancing is sometimes the best alternative. When you feel you are losing control, get away from the battle zone and regroup.

Coping With Patients Who Refuse Treatment

If a patient refuses a diagnostic procedure or some form of therapy, find out why. Noncompliance often revolves around a lack of joint agreement on goals. Does the patient understand what is going to be done and why? The hidden message of a depressed person may be "what is the use?"[7]

When a refusal takes place, reaffirm the patient's right to do so. Once patients are reassured that they do indeed have some control over their care, they become less defensive and antagonistic. You are perceived as an advocate rather than an adversary.

The next step is to get the patient to reconsider his decision. Simply asking the patient what he thinks should be done may provide the solution. In some situations, this persuasion should be undertaken by the attending physician who explains the purpose of the diagnostic or therapeutic procedure and exactly what it comprises.

In most instances, the combination of advocacy and clarification will do the trick. If not, encourage the patient to ask still more questions. Despite your best efforts, he still may not have understood what is going on.

NEVER ARGUE. If you fail, enlist the aid of a behavioral specialist, the most persuasive member of the medical team, the caregiver who has the best rapport with the patient, or a family member.

REFERENCES

1. Ritvo MM. Who are the "good" and "bad" patients? *Mod Hosp.* 1963;100:79-81.

2. Herbert CP, Seifert MH Jr. When the patient is the problem. *Patient Care.* 1990;24:59-76.

3. Montgomery CL. Patients are more than customers. *Am J Nursing.* 1988;88:1257-1258.

4. Luna ML. The patient who complains. *Nursing.* 1984;14:47-49.

5. Cox HC. Verbal abuse in nursing. *Nursing Manage.* 1987;18:47-50.

6. Hobbs T. You can change a patient's problem behavior. *Nursing Life.* 1983;3:44-49.

7. Laken DD. Protecting patients against themselves: what to do when patients refuse treatment. *Nursing.* 1983;13:90-94.

16. Difficult Bosses

Your ability to establish a mutually valuable relationship with your boss is, and will continue to be, a major factor in determining your success or failure at work."[1]

Sooner or later, most employees find themselves working for a superior whom they regard as intolerable. Some bosses can be described as rigid, authoritarian, overpaid, self-serving, and overrated, but most of them are decent people, devoted to getting their jobs done effectively. They are human beings with strengths and weaknesses just like everybody else.[1]

Specific charges against superiors include every kind of possible vexatious behavior discussed—unethical, immoral, or illegal acts, petty annoyances, hostility—you name it. When the difficult person is the boss, the problem escalates because of the power, or perceived power, of that person. Because of this, subordinates are ill-advised to respond to bosses the same way they might respond to their colleagues.

Bosses are often not aware of the stress they cause or the self-esteem they decimate. The more intolerable they become, the less likely they are to get feedback from the targets of their irksome actions. The employees may fear the repercussions of any complaints on their part about boss-induced stress. When they do speak up, they will direct their charges at upper management or general working conditions rather than at their immediate superior. The absence of such feedback reduces the likelihood that these leaders will change their offending behavior.

Dissatisfied subordinates with spunk simply depart, leaving the boss surrounded by sycophants and spiritless passive workers. The tyrants who are cognizant of the damage they inflict but do not try to change their ways are even worse because they take a sadistic satisfaction from their behavior.

SELECT A GOOD BOSS

When you are considering a position change, the reputation of the person to whom you will report should be one of the most important factors to consider. Only if you are desperate, or you know that the manager is leaving soon, should you accept a job when you learn that the person in charge makes life miserable for her associates.

A little probing can quickly provide such information. Insist on talking to some of the current employees or, still better, one who has recently resigned. Inquire about the rate of turnover in the department. During your employment interview, ask penetrating questions that reveal the manager's leadership style.

ACCEPT RESPONSIBILITY FOR THE RELATIONSHIP

We have a perfect right to evaluate our relationship with our leaders, but we should be hesitant to judge them. When we say, "My boss is an incompetent communicator," we are judging. Our subjective conclusion about our boss' competency may or may not be correct. More importantly, we are placing all the blame on her, absolving ourselves of any responsibility. However, when we say, "My boss and I have difficulty communicating. We frequently end up yelling at each other," we are not judging the boss, we are evaluating the relationship. In addition, we are admitting that maybe we are partly responsible for the communication problem.

We have limited control over our boss' behavior, but we have complete control over how we react to it. It is not necessary that you like your boss or that she like you. It is only necessary that you do not dislike each other to a degree that prevents treating each other with respect and courtesy and discharging each of your responsibilities. Bosses with low self-esteem are difficult to work for; employees with low self-esteem are hard to manage.[1] Therefore, it is in the best interest of both the boss and the employee to work toward enhancing and preserving each other's self-esteem (see chapter 3).

BE LOYAL

The cardinal rule of loyalty is to make one's leader look good. It is easy to support the boss in her presence, but it is so tempting to join the critics when she is not around. Individuals who continually bad-mouth their superiors undermine their own reputations. Observers cannot help but conclude that if the critics had anything on the ball, they would not stick with such an intolerable superior.

Giving the boss credit for ideas and support is loyalty in action. Giving the boss credit she does not deserve is manipulation that will eventually backfire.

If you try to circumvent your boss by bypassing her, your loyalty will be questioned. The end-run strategy is to go over your boss' head to report or complain to her superior. Resort to this only in critical situations, such as sexual harassment by your boss or when you are ready to resign. In other cases, however, what you perceive as mistreatment and leads to your urge to go over the boss' head may be based on a false assumption. For example:

Alice, your boss, turned down your request to attend an important professional meeting. You had already registered for this meeting, and your plane tickets were on your desk. Then, Alice approved a similar request from one of your colleagues. You were furious, and you understandably felt that she had demonstrated favoritism and you were justified in going to Steve, Alice's boss, to complain. Your better judgment led you to go to Alice first. At that meeting, you learned that Alice wanted to send you, but she was overruled by Steve. Alice was too upset to talk to you about this at the time.

When you have a complaint about your boss, confront her in a quiet, respectful way. Focus on the facts and give her ample chance to respond. Never lose your cool.

Often, behaviors such as being on time for staff meetings, showing up for departmental social events, being willing to work overtime, or exhibiting enthusiasm and optimism are interpreted by managers as evidence of loyalty.

Keep your boss informed. If one of your boss' superiors talks directly to you about anything—anything at all—go to your boss immediately after that meeting and repeat what transpired. Insecure managers are especially grateful for this information.

Try to deliver glad tidings, but do not hide bad news, even when it relates to a mistake you made, and do not blame others for those errors. On the other hand, do not accept the blame for other people's goofs unless they report to you. If you are blamed for something that is not your fault, do not make a big fuss about it while your boss is still hot under the collar. Come back later and explain things in a polite, straightforward manner.

Do not annoy your boss with trivia. When you bring the boss problems, always have one or more suggestions for solving those problems. Avoid even using the word "problem." Instead of, "Mary, we have a problem," say, "Mary, we have an opportunity for an improvement. Here is what I have in mind."[2]

Empathize. Invest a little time in trying to see work situations from the boss' perspective. Encourage the boss to vent her feelings, and be certain to honor confidentiality.

Help the boss to cope with her deficiencies. For example, if your boss hates to give verbal presentations or to prepare complicated reports, offer to substitute at meetings and to prepare rough drafts of reports. Start right now by identifying three ways you can be more valuable to the person to whom you report.

PREVENT PROBLEMS

Analyze your temperament and that of your boss (see chapter 12). Use that knowledge to readjust your attitude and interpersonal relationships. Adapt your communication style to that of your boss. If your boss prefers one-on-one verbal messages, talk to her directly instead of sending notes and reports. If the boss issues numerous memos and letters and seems impatient when you want to talk, keep your word processor busy. If the boss is kinesthetically inclined, use a lot of handshaking, touching, and verbal expressions such as, "I feel that..." or "I just cannot handle that...."

Be cordial with secretaries and administrative assistants. They can increase your awareness of how the boss operates, including the boss' likes and dislikes. They can expedite or delay your reports and even influence the boss' evaluation of your performance. Many talented employees have been derailed because they did not get along with (or became too familiar with) these key people.

If you want to be treated as a professional, then look and act like one. Make yourself needed but do not do anything that would lead your boss to see you as a threat.

Compliment, but do not flatter. Praise must be sincere, believable, and not overdone. Use "third-person praising" (praising when the recipients are not present). These compliments will get back to the boss, and you are less likely to be classified as an apple-polisher.

HANDLING PROBLEM BOSSES

There are three responses to impossible bosses:

1. Change them (not often viable)
2. Leave them (only as the last resort)
3. Change your attitude and behavior toward them (usually best)

Catch the boss doing something right and reinforce that behavior by praising or thanking her for it. For example:

"Dr. Johnson, in the past we have been disturbed by how some physicians blame us for things that are beyond our control—and no one in the department defends us. But today, when you came storming out of your office and told Dr. Adams that she was off base, we all silently applauded."

For your own peace of mind, better time management, and greater effectiveness, learn how to say no to the boss in a tactful and respectful manner. Never say, "I do not want to," "That is your job," or "I was not hired to do that." Explain why you must refuse or object. Do not give phony excuses. Instead, offer alternatives—say what you will do.

Following are some common problem bosses and helpful tips for coping with them and their difficult behaviors.

The New Bosses

Getting a new boss is like starting a new job. Be ready to adopt to new ways of doing things. Adapt your work style to that of the new leader. Pay attention to the new boss' statements about what she likes and dislikes. Let her know what support you need. Do everything you can to help the boss adjust. If you had your differences with your previous superior, do not bad-mouth that person. Instead, regard this as an opportunity to get off to a good new start.

The Bosses Who Need to be Liked

When bosses have an intense need to be liked, they are rarely successful in the long haul. These individuals are very sociable and likable. They smile a lot and agree with everything that anybody says. They are often called wimps or ultra-agreeables because they cannot say no. Some of their colleagues and associates will take advantage of these bosses, and the morale of the other employees then plummets.

These managers either lack courage or fail to realize that respect is more important than popularity. Because they do not earn respect, they do not and cannot follow through on their promises. They rarely take risks and are inveterate buck passers—constantly calling meetings, asking opinions, and running things by the top brass.

Solution: Help these managers by confronting them with candid statements about how the team would function better if they were stronger and less concerned about popularity.[1] Praise them when they show some backbone. Offer to serve as gatekeeper when it comes to making requests, standing up to outsiders, and defending turf. If you or your department are constantly stressed because your boss makes promises that cannot be fulfilled, your only ultimate decision may be to leave.

The Con Artists

Like the bosses who need to be liked, the con artists promise a lot but deliver little or only insignificant favors. However, unlike the wimps, they do not lack courage or have a compulsion for friendship. They are expert manipulators who have a selfish motivation.

Solution: Do not trust or rely on these devious people. Think carefully before you make commitments. Try to ferret out what they really are after. Do not threaten them by accusations of manipulation or put them on the defensive.[3]

The Overdelegators

Bosses who are overdelegators prove that there can always be too much of a good thing. While it is a good general policy to accept delegated tasks, especially those that are career developers, you can become overwhelmed.

Solution: If your regular assignments are starting to suffer, ask your boss to establish priorities or to relieve you of some of the work. You may be able to delegate some of the work to one of your associates. At times you must say no or accept assignments conditionally.

The Laissez-faire Leaders

Laissez-faire (also called "hands-off" or "free-rein") leaders abdicate much of their power. They give little direction and allow their employees a great deal of freedom. While this style is appropriate in certain situations, such as in a research laboratory where the workers are highly skilled and independent thinkers, problems develop in the usual work arena when employees need advice, guidance, and support. Many professionals, however, prefer this type of leader to the autocratic type.

Solution: Determine what your authority is and use it. Revise your position description to include more control over your areas of responsibility. Seek broad approval for your objectives, plans, and schedules, then go ahead with them. Pin the boss down when she issues vague directives. Gradually assume more responsibility and control.

The Stallers and Procrastinators

Stallers and procrastinators always need more data or have to check with their superiors. They busy themselves with trivia because they cannot face up to the important tasks and decisions.

Solution: When you want an approval, have all the data ready. Reassure your boss that you have checked your proposal out with the experts. Be optimistic. Try to find the reasons for her hesitancy and eliminate them. Establish deadlines for her approval and give reasons for these target dates. Force the issue by a statement such as, "If I do not hear from you by Friday, I will go ahead, okay?" As much as possible, keep the action steps under your control.

The Unfair Bosses

Unfair bosses play favorites or may even violate laws against discrimination. Some favoritism is evident in most worksites, and most of the time it is not a big deal. However, employees have the right to object when blatant differences exist with regard to access to the boss, assignments, advancement, pay, educational opportunities, schedules, and promotions.

Solution: It is beyond the scope of this book to elaborate on the ramifications of the various laws against discrimination and formal complaints handled via union contracts. Suffice it to say that if anyone feels that illegal discrimination is taking place, that person should report it. In chapter 25 we discuss sexual harassment at some length.

In some cases of favoritism, the group leader is not aware of how her actions are being perceived by team members. If approached tactfully by a group of employees, she may modify her interpersonal relationships for the better. Avoid being the only person to make such accusations. When the favoritism is based on nepotism, it is usually best to ask for a transfer or to look for a new employer.

The Fire-fighters

Fire-fighters practice management-by-crisis. They eschew managing-by-wandering-around and instead can usually be found in their offices where they wait until people bring them problems. Problems coming into the boss' office are bigger than those detected at workstations because they have been allowed to develop into crises. They are harder to resolve and are seldom completely reversible. Fire-fighters are disasters when it comes to planning, deadlines, and proactive leadership.

Solution: When you see a problem developing in your area, alert the fire-fighter. If she chooses to ignore your warning, then that decision is her responsibility. Try to avoid assignments in which your leader should be exerting more direction, but then blames the person doing the work when things go awry. Stay out of the fire-fighter's way when she emerges from her office with all the bells and whistles blaring.

The Reverse End-runners

The downward communication of reverse end-runners (people who are above you in the organizational hierarchy) does not follow the chain of command. Reverse end-runners give orders to your employees without your knowledge. This puts your staffers on the spot, especially when the orders are contrary to the ones you have issued.

Generally, these bosses do this not to undermine your authority but simply because you were not on the scene at the time. For example: Sara, a supervisor in the radiology department, finds that in her absence one of the radiologists often rearranges the daily schedule without consulting her. Usually, the radiologist has no valid reasons for changing the schedule. Furthermore, the radiologist failed to tell Sara that she had made the changes, thus resulting in confusion between the radiology department and the floor nurse supervisors.

Solution: When your boss often bypasses you, consider why she does it. Usually, the best remedy is to sit down and discuss the matter with her. Use specific examples to show how the interference causes loss of efficiency, confuses your staff, and undermines your authority.

Here are some more tips for minimizing this problem:

1. Authorize your staffers to make certain decisions when orders conflict. Consider efficiency, customer satisfaction, and the importance of employees feeling that they have control of their work.

2. Make a list of services that can be modified by other people and who those other people are. For example, in the pathology laboratory, each pathologist may select modifications in tissue staining procedures.

3. Provide a list of services or procedures that may not be modified without your specific approval. Train your subordinates on how to respond courteously to requests that are not to be honored. For example, they should not say what they may not do, but only what they can do: "I can draw the blood specimen right now and will ask my supervisor if we can do the test this morning," not "We never do those tests in the morning." An alternative is for your employees to diplomatically refer unusual requests or demands to you.

The Bureaucrats

These follow-the-book bosses thrive in large governmental organizations where they can take refuge behind policies, rules, and memos from upper management. The policy manual is their bible. They lack flexibility and avoid risks like the plague. Today's technical and organizational changes provide a hostile environment for these leaders. They do not adjust well to change, and the result is that they become as obsolescent as their methods. When you return to their hospital after some time, you find that their units have been moved to the basement or some other out-of-the-way location. Their staffs and their responsibility are reduced. If this type of leadership characterizes the entire organization, that organization may not survive the 90s.

Solution: If you work in a very stable unit and have little or no desire to move up in the organization, you may enjoy working for a bureaucrat. It can be very comfortable. But if you want to be part of the leading edge of health care, look for a new leader.

The Tyrants

These empire builders care only about getting more power, turf, and subordinates. Their loyalty to people and to their employers is minimal. They want complete control over everything and crush anyone who stands in their way. They are arrogant, abrasive, and demeaning. Their win-lose attitude is repeatedly expressed as, "I am right; you are wrong."

Solution: Appear firm, strong, and unemotional. Let them rage; do not back up, cringe, or cry. Never tell them they are wrong. Do not counterpunch. When you want approval for something, illustrate how it will benefit the boss. Suggested verbal responses include the following[4]:

> "When you say insulting things like that, how do you think that makes us feel?"
> "I can see that you do not agree, but it would seem that...."
> "Excuse me, I am not through."

The Bosses With Alcohol or Drug Problems

Bosses with alcohol or drug problems bring grief to their colleagues, subordinates, management, family members, and themselves. When under the influence of these addictive substances, they may become abusive or irritable or exercise poor judgment. All too often, other members of their team cover for them, so the problem persists much too long.

Solution: Here are Quick's[5] common-sense recommendations for supporting members of the work group:

1. Learn their drinking or drug abuse patterns and take damage control measures. For example, if the boss has long martini lunches, hold up any reports that she must approve until the next morning.
2. Do not join the drinkers. They often like company.

3. Do not get emotionally involved.
4. Do not pretend that there is no problem.
5. Learn how much authority you have when she is absent—which is probably often.
6. Do not stay on board too long unless the boss gets medical help.

I would add to Quick's list that if the leader's drug or alcohol problem poses a threat to the safety or welfare of patients or employees, the problem should be reported to the personnel department or to the boss' superior.

The Bosses Who Perceive You as a Threat

The more experienced and competent you are, and the more insecure and incompetent your boss is, the greater is the risk that you will be perceived as a threat.

Solution: Minimize the threat by keeping your boss informed, praising her strengths, and not seeking recognition for yourself. Ask her opinion and thank her profusely for it. Do not exceed your authority. Never point out the boss' deficiencies to others. It will get back to the boss and then you are really in the doghouse. This does not mean, however, that you should become a doormat. If you perform competently, others will notice your good work and comment about it. Submit reports (via the boss) up the chain of command. Take opportunities to make presentations at meetings and to serve on cross-functional committees.

When you have serious differences of opinion with the boss, express them, but do most of this in private. When you disagree in public, do it tactfully. If you handle the situation well, your boss will eventually perceive you as an ally rather than as a threat.

Working for Two Bosses

Many people now report to two bosses. Reductions-in-force (RIFs) often result in a secretary serving more than one executive. In the laboratory, a tissue technologist may report both to a pathologist and a laboratory manager or chief medical technologist. Pleasing both bosses can be difficult. Deadlines and priorities are frequently the bones of contention.

Solution: Diplomatically confront the junior person and encourage that manager to modify her demands or expectations. At other times, it is better to talk to both managers separately or together. Be diplomatic and show that you are anxious to please both bosses. Offer specific solutions, such as assigning one of your staff members to each manager. Summarize whatever agreement is reached, and thank them for cooperating.[6]

Other common boss problems are described in subsequent chapters:
Unethical Bosses—Chapter 20
Know-it-alls—Chapter 23
Hostile Bosses—Chapter 24
Sexual Harassers—Chapter 25
Workaholics—Chapter 27

REFERENCES

1. Hegarty C. *How to Manage Your Boss*. Mill Valley, Calif: Whatever Publishing Co; 1982.
2. Bernstein AJ, Rozen SC. *Dinosaur Brains: Dealing With All Those Impossible People at Work*. New York, NY: John Wiley & Sons; 1989.
3. Krupar K, Krupar JJ. Jerks at work. *Personnel J*. 1988;67:68-74.
4. Solomon M. *Working With Difficult People*. Englewood Cliffs, NJ: Prentice Hall; 1990.
5. Quick TL. *Managing People at Work*. New York, NY: Executive Enterprises Publishers; 1987.
6. Knippen JY, Green TB, Sutton KH. How to handle problems with two bosses. *Supervis Manage*. August 1991:9.

17. The Underperformers

U nderperformers are employees whose productivity or accuracy is not up to the expectations of their superiors. Productivity is not the only thing that suffers when one or more employees do not carry their share of the workload. Teamwork also suffers because the other employees resent having to carry the "deadwood." The situation deteriorates still more when supervisors accept the unsatisfactory results and even make excuses for the underperformers.

Disappointing workers fall into two major categories: those who never performed up to expectations and those whose work slipped after months or years of adequate or outstanding performance.

THE NINE MAJOR CAUSES OF UNDERPERFORMANCE

Absence of Work Standards

Employees are disciplined when their work does not adhere to policies, rules, and regulations; employees are considered to be underperformers when their work does not meet expected standards. Policies and other behavioral guidelines are spelled out in employee handbooks; performance standards are described in position descriptions. A charge of underperformance must be based on established work standards. These standards should not be based on the levels performed by superior or even average workers. They must represent the minimal level that is acceptable.

Unfortunately, these performance criteria are often ill-defined or ignored. Our employees do not have the bells and buzzers that are built into automated instruments. As supervisors, we may pay more attention to the performance of our instruments than we do to that of our employees.

Work standards are especially important when new positions are created because the performance of the incumbent cannot be compared and contrasted with that of previous workers. The expectations of supervisors are expressed in position descriptions and performance standards, and the latter are emphasized during the orientation and training of new hires. When these standards clearly represent what is expected, the employee does not require as much verbal feedback to know how well he is performing. Also, surprises are less likely to occur when he receives his performance ratings.

Employees Just Cannot Do Any Better

Some employees are simply not qualified for their positions. They know what they must do, but they could not do it if their life depended on it, despite all your training and support. They should not have been hired in the first place. In chapter 5, we discussed the importance of selecting people who are less likely to be problems. This holds true for underperformers. Careful screening will exclude the more obvious risks.

If you do hire an employee who is unqualified, chalk this experience up to an error in the personnel selection process. Change the job or the job holder. All too often, supervisors try to give such employees special consideration and keep them beyond their probationary periods. This is bad for the supervisor, bad for the company, and especially bad for the unfortunate employee who by this time is perfectly miserable in the job.

Employees Do Not Know the Significance of What They Do

If employees fail to see how their job fits into the goals of the organization, they lack the interest and motivation needed to perform well. Without the "big picture" perspective on things, they become automatons churning out their dreary task day after day without realizing the importance of their work. For example, Jeffrey spends most of the day preparing and staining cytology smears for the cytotechnologists. His interest and performance increased when one of the cytotechs took the time to explain how the quality of the smears affected the accuracy of cancer diagnosis and how he could improve the technical quality of the smears.

Absence of Feedback

Although employees may have received some negative off-the-cuff comments from their superiors, they have not learned that their work has been substandard. Without this feedback, they continue to perform inadequately.

External Obstacles

External obstacles to work performance include: adverse work environment (temperature, humidity, odors, lighting, noise); substandard facilities (physical layouts, equipment, supplies); inappropriate work-flow patterns; inadequate rewards (salary, raises, bonuses, promotions, recognition); excessive red tape (policies, rules, procedures); poor supervision; and disgruntled associates. Supervisors must be particularly sensitive to the particular physical needs of their employees. Eliminate from the workplace any safety hazards that may cause accidents.

Internal Obstacles

Internal or personal obstacles include absence of satisfaction with the work itself, low self-esteem, feeling of powerlessness, poor health, and emotional, financial, family, or substance abuse problems.

Good Performance is Not Rewarded or is Penalized

Many supervisors have a bad habit of overloading their high performers with extra work. Unless the additional assignments are tasks that these employees enjoy, they will feel that their good performance is being punished. This inference is supported by their observations that the chronic complainers in the department receive lighter work loads and are rarely asked to do anything extra. Often, employees who perform well may be sensitive to the reaction of coworkers who either do not live up to the same standards or who respond negatively to their above-average work. For example:

■ Julie, a new employee, follows to the letter every safety rule and preventive medical precaution. Her vigilance begins to slip, however, when she sees senior professionals violating these same rules and precautions.

■ Jack, out on the hospital loading dock, worked hard and without complaint until his buddies start calling him a "rate-buster" and shunning him. Now he takes his time and joins in the griping.

■ Good performance is punished in other ways as well. Louise, who heads up a hospital medical records department, was ecstatic when she received the plaudits of the comptroller for keeping her department's expenditures under budget for the past year. Those good feelings vanished when Louise discovered that her budget for the next year was slashed by the amount that she had saved.

Behavioral psychologists agree that the kind of performance you want must be reinforced by rewards, especially recognition and praise. Failure to do so results in performance decline, except for those few self-motivators who get such immense satisfaction from their work that they do not need any external stimuli.

Poor Performance is Rewarded

At times, supervisors inadvertently reward poor performance. Employees may exhibit inappropriate behavior that is intended to "get a rise out of" the boss. When the boss reacts, the underperformer's mission is accomplished. For example:

■ Alice often skips departmental meetings without legitimate excuses. When she does show up, she saunters in casually and without apologizing. Her supervisor, who has a thing about attendance, periodically chews Alice out, sometimes in front of the group. But Alice seems to enjoy her notoriety. It is the only time she gets any attention from her supervisor, and her rebellious behavior is secretly admired by her coworkers.

Across-the-board salary increases, without regard for performance, perpetuate marginal or low productivity. Avoid giving bonuses or salary increases to people who are performing marginally, and be certain to document deficiencies and counseling sessions. For example:

■ Supervisor Sam received several special pay raises because he was the only person in his department who could keep the computer from "crashing." Sam periodically threatens to take his skill to a competitor. Sam has several intelligent associates who could learn to troubleshoot the apparatus, but Sam always has an excuse for not training them. When challenged, he responds with, "You know what happened last time I tried to do that." No one knows what that mysterious misadventure was or who was involved. Sam just shakes his head and walks away.

Supervisors may also unknowingly allow employees to avoid taking on other challenges by relying too much on their tried-and-true abilities. For example:

■ Sue, a senior operating room technologist, is still helping Dr. Jones do his hemorrhoidectomies. Sue enjoys assisting with this simple operation and listening to his unending stream of funny stories that punctuate the operation. When the operating room supervisor tries to schedule Sue to help with more complex surgical procedures, Sue gets Dr. Jones to demand her services, and she gets away with it.

Employees Do Not Want to Do Any Better

At times, employees lose their desire to excel and get stuck in a rut of mediocrity. For example:

■ Ron likes things the way they are. He performs the minimum requirements for his position but still has time to relax at work. He enjoys a high reward/risk ratio. His reward is socializing with colleagues, and no risk has been apparent to him up to this point. Ron's boss just shakes his head and tells you that Ron has an attitude problem. That seems to excuse Ron's boss from any responsibility—or so he thinks.

When a supervisor thinks that an employee like Ron is just plain lazy, has a poor work ethic, or has some other attitudinal problem, that supervisor should look for answers to the following questions: What are Ron's goals, and how does Ron perceive his job? Does he find the work demeaning or monotonous? Boring, monotonous work done by overqualified people is a major source of underperformance. How is his health? Could his energy level be low because of poor health? If he has a history of frequent job changes, why has he been a job-hopper?

Ron's boss should show personal interest in Ron, learn more about his family and social activities, point out that he is letting the team down, or pair him up with a hard worker. Ron's opinion should be solicited once in a while, or he could be involved in some problem solving. Recognition and praise may be effective. Ron may need retraining or cross-training. His motivation might increase if he became a local expert in something that would increase his prestige. Ron eventually did become a hard worker when he received special training in AIDS and started giving a series of lectures on this subject to student nurses and colleagues.

THE TYPES OF UNDERPERFORMERS

Underperformers come in many shapes and sizes. The key to coping with these difficult employees is to find out the underlying causes of their underperformance and to take proactive measures to address them.

Passed-over Employees

Sally lost out on a promotion. Now she is less productive and has become stridently critical of the administration. Her former teammate, Bruce, who won the promotion, now has to deal with Sally.

Bruce can try to get Sally to serve as an advisor and back-up. He could give Sally some choice assignments and delegate some administrative responsibilities to her. If Sally remains resentful and obstructive, Bruce will have to hold a frank dialogue with her, stating exactly what he will and will not tolerate and what he expects in the future.

Spurt Workers

Most departments have at least one person who only works hard in spurts. He may often outperform other colleagues, but only when he applies himself. Like the hare in the old tortoise-and-hare story, these employees waste time in between spurts of hard work, so that even though their total work accomplishments are satisfactory, they set a bad example for others.

Sometimes it is best for supervisors to do nothing. However, when these individuals waste other people's time or are seen performing nonwork activities, such as balancing their checkbooks or tying up a telephone with personal calls, they force your hand.

Giving these hot-and-cold performers additional assignments and more challenging tasks is usually more effective than admonishing them about wasting time. The latter approach usually gets the same kind of response you get from people who arrive late and/or leave early: "I get my work done, don't I?" If that scenario develops, explain how their nonwork activities affect other employees. At counseling sessions, encourage these spurt workers to eliminate some of their time-wasting habits. For example, they should ask their friends and relatives to call them at home instead of at work.

A good time to increase their workload or responsibility is when one of their fellow workers leaves. At that time, you can shift some of the departing person's work to the spurt worker. You can also give him the responsibility for helping to train the replacement.

Slow Workers

Some people just poke along at a slow pace. If you mention their low productivity, they will usually brush it off with a comment about how their work is done more carefully and that "haste makes waste." Other workers may slow down because of poor health, low energy levels, inability to adjust to changes in assignments or staffing, loss of interest, or frustration over their rank in the organization. Workers who lack motivation may divert their attention to outside interests rather than focusing on the job at hand.

Here are some suggestions for handling these slowpokes:

1. Do not criticize them until you have done everything you can to show them how to work more efficiently.
2. Let them know that there is a problem and what your productivity standards are.
3. Set deadlines and priorities.
4. Send them to seminars on time management.

Perfectionists

Perfectionists are not slow workers, they just do not get a lot done because they feel that they must do every task, no matter how small, exactly right. They insist on eliminating error by repeating or double-checking everything. They often become bottlenecks in the flow of work. If you insist that they work faster, they will make an error sooner or later and then trap you into the psychological game of "see what you made me do."

Perfectionists have difficulty getting along with their peers, who they accuse of sloppy performance.[1] They are very hard on subordinates, demanding that same degree of perfectionism.

Handling these people takes loads of patience. Find work slots for them where their delays do not clog major workflow channels. Assign them tasks that do require a high degree of accuracy. In immunohematology labs, for example, they are great at investigating the causes of transfusion reactions.

In the legal or finance department, they are right at home making the final check of important contracts or budgets. You may be able to speed them up a little by holding them to deadlines.

Time Wasters

The most common forms of time wasting are tardiness, early departures from work, excessive socializing, personal phone calls, and abuses of sick leave. The following measures can help control these time thefts:

1. Emphasize good work habits during orientation.
2. Set a good example.
3. Develop flexible work schedules.
4. Avoid overstaffing.
5. Teach employees how to keep busy when waiting for further instructions.
6. Provide backup assignments to fill spare time.
7. Counsel and/or discipline chronic offenders.

Unmotivated Employees

If workers lose motivation, their performance suffers. Steps can be taken, however, to recharge their tired batteries. Retraining may become necessary as jobs and technology change. The saying, "You can't teach an old dog a new trick" has been proven false time and again. Send employees to workshops or seminars. Even the most unmotivated workers return from these meetings with renewed interest in their field.

You may be able to rekindle unmotivated employees' interests by assigning trainees to them. A sense of purpose is important, and many people find the role of counselor, mentor, or teacher to be enriching.[2] Take advantage of your seasoned employees' experience and technical know-how, but be careful—you do not want negative attitudes rubbing off onto the newcomers.

Plateaued Employees

Plateaued employees are those who reach their promotional ceiling long before they retire.[3] Do not confuse plateauing with the Peter principle— plateaued employees have not risen to their level of incompetence. They are competent in their positions, but they are not capable of going beyond it.

Responses to plateauing vary markedly. For some, it represents a tender trap. They may continue to contribute eagerly. Others quit and leave. Still others "quit" and stay but ooze resentment or frustration. Most plateaued employees fall between these extremes.

The following executive actions are effective when dealing with plateaued employees:

1. Minimize the number of people caught in this trap by developing dual career ladders or increasing the number of rungs in the ladder.
2. Transfer, discharge, or encourage early retirement.
3. Create "minipromotions" by flattening the hierarchical pyramid (ie, reducing the number of managers). In the resulting more "horizontal" organization, all employees including the plateaued ones must assume more responsibility.
4. Expand their educational opportunities.
5. Award title changes that promote self-worth.

Convert plateaued employees from hand-wringers into risk-takers.[4] The following supervisory measures help to keep enthusiasm alive. They also signal that the organization still values the work of these employees.

1. Watch for signs of mental cruise control: "I just want to do my job and go home."
2. Provide more training. Consider staff rotation and cross-training.
3. Find ways to enrich their jobs. Assign them to project teams. Encourage innovation; get them to use their knowledge in new ways.
4. Consult with the person on problems and operational aspects of your department. Ask for advice. These people have a great deal of practical experience.[5]
5. Give them additional authority or more control over their activities. Freedom and flexibility may be seen as recognition for past experience and contributions. Delegate special one-time assignments.[5]
6. Use the employee as a teacher. The experienced person may be valuable in one-on-one situations, helping to orient new employees or teaching present ones new procedures.[5]
7. Get them to analyze their past successes and setbacks, taking the best from both, and building on a strong foundation.
8. Seek concurrence on new goals.
9. Encourage them to expand their networks. Point the plateaued employee toward certain prestige assignments such as committee work, attendance at seminars, or the coordination of a social activity.
10. Boost self-esteem through more recognition, praise, involvement in planning, and decision making.

A caveat: The plateaued employee takes criticism badly because it is a threat to his standing. Being critical or threatening toward him will not succeed in improving performance.

REFERENCES

1. Bernstein AJ, Rozen SC. *Dinosaur Brains: Dealing With All Those Impossible People at Work*. New York, NY: John Wiley & Sons; 1989.
2. Hagen RP. Older workers: how to utilize this valuable resource. *Supervis Manage*. 1983;28:2-9.
3. Bardwick JM. *The Plateauing Trap*. New York, NY: AMACOM; 1987.
4. Kaye B. Are plateaued performers productive? *Personnel J*. 1991;68:56-65.
5. McConnell CR. *The Effective Health Care Supervisor*. Rockville, Md: Aspen Publishing Co; 1988.

18.   Employees Who Do Not Show Up

Sorry, boss, but I cannot make it in today." Practically every supervisor has had multiple battles with absenteeism. Just when a problem appears to be under control, another fire breaks out.

Absenteeism is such a common and serious problem that it merits its own chapter, even though the proactive and reactive solutions are basically the same as for other behavioral problems. The methods discussed in the chapters on coaching, counseling, and disciplining hold true for the attendance problem.

Unexcused absence is the single most common disciplinary problem in the United States.[1] On any given day, about one million American workers fail to show up for work. Some are sick, but many do not show up just because they do not feel like it. Fortunately, most workers come to work even when they are indisposed simply because of a sense of loyalty to their employer or their fellow workers.

Absenteeism negatively impacts productivity, quality, profitability, and morale. While it cannot be eliminated, it can be controlled by identifying and eliminating its causes, establishing and implementing control programs, and practicing competent supervision.[2]

MEASURES OF ABSENTEEISM

The following formulas can measure absenteeism:

1.   Percentage of absences: Number of days absent, divided by number of work days during study period, multiplied by 100.

2. Proportion of absence episodes: Number of absence episodes of any length, divided by number of days scheduled for work during study period, multiplied by 100.
3. Proportion of 1- to 2-day absence episodes: Number of 1- to 2-day absence episodes, divided by number of days scheduled for work during study period, multiplied by 100.

Why do employees not show up? Many work and personal factors influence an employee's decision to attend work or to stay away. Most industrial behaviorists agree that satisfying work, sound group relationships, people-oriented leadership styles, and a positive work ethic encourage employee attendance.[3]

The presence of work dissatisfiers or the absence of motivators cuts into job attendance. Negative factors of major significance are perceptions of inadequate pay, dull or monotonous tasks, lack of opportunity for growth, and a feeling of being taken for granted.

When supervisors are unpopular or autocratic, absenteeism represents a way for employees to strike back. A vicious cycle ensues. The supervisors get tougher and tougher about attendance; the employees take more and more time off.

TRADITIONAL METHODS FOR COPING WITH ABSENTEEISM

Discipline is still the most commonly used measure for coping with absenteeism, despite reports that organizations using this as their only control method have higher-than-average absence rates.[4]

Some employers require a physician's certification of illness for absences beyond a set limit. This is both ineffective and inconvenient for everyone involved. It rarely works, except to determine if the employee is medically able to return to her job.

Another negative approach is to dock the pay of employees who do not telephone their supervisors by midmorning of the day of absence. This unfairly penalizes workers who have legitimate excuses for failing to notify their bosses. It also does not appease the employee's peers who still have to do the absent employee's work.

Reducing the number of paid sick days increases attendance. Studies show a direct correlation between the number of allowable absences and the rate of absenteeism. According to the Bureau of Labor Statistics, government workers use almost twice as many sick days as retail trade employees, since in retail, if you do not work, sometimes you do not get paid.[5]

Bribes for showing up do not always work. General Motors spent over $400 million in bonuses for employees who used less sick leave. This strategy did not affect the overall rate of absenteeism.[1] Other reward systems include payment for any unused sick leave at year-end, permitted accrual of vacation and sick leave, or additional days off. Most carrot-or-stick approaches are not effective, at least over the long haul.

Other schemes include awarding extra vacation days for perfect attendance for a period of time, such as 6 months. Another is to give chances in lotteries to people with perfect records.

One of the more effective strategies is the so-called "no-fault" or "point" system.[6] With this method, there are no excused or unexcused absences, just absences. Employees need not justify them. Employees are entitled to a limited number of points (paid absences) each year.

Each absence, regardless of length, is recorded as one occurrence. For example, if a worker is absent on Monday and Friday, she is charged with two absences; but if that worker is absent all week, that counts as only one occurrence. This system avoids penalizing employees who are really sick and must be absent for several days. It sticks it to the ones who fail to show up on Mondays, Fridays, days before or after holidays, or on the day after pay day.

A potential disadvantage of this strategy is that employees may abuse the system by staying home for more than one day since a series of days counts the same as a single day's absence. However, companies that have used this system have not found this type of abuse to be a problem. In fact, another advantage of such a program is that people who are still feeling poorly, but who want to minimize their use of paid sick days, will now stay home rather than returning too soon and bringing contagious illnesses with them or not performing safely or efficiently on the job.

ROLE OF UPPER MANAGEMENT

Overall attendance throughout an organization is usually within acceptable limits when the quality of work life is high. When employers provide what workers regard as satisfactory compensation and working conditions, they will come to work. When the employees are proud to work for an organization, attendance rates soar.

Actions can often be taken to make it easier for people to come to work. The formation of car pools may overcome transportation difficulties. Flexible work hours and day-care for children and older parents decrease the need to feign illness to take care of personal matters.

The availability on the worksite of enthusiastic medical and nursing staffs can help workers who are not feeling well decide to come to work or to finish a workday. When an employee who is not feeling well can drop into the medical clinic and receive relief and advice, she is less likely to ask for the rest of the day off. For the same reason, she is less likely to stay at home for minor complaints. The availability of this service may eliminate the need for expensive physician office visits, and employees appreciate that. Supervisors appreciate the advice of clinic personnel in making decisions as to when an employee should remain on the job or be permitted to return after an illness.

ROLE OF SUPERVISORS

Supervisors have three major roles in controlling chronic absenteeism. In descending order of importance these are:

1. Good leadership—the proactive approach.
2. Interpret, promulgate, and enforce polices pertaining to attendance.
3. Counsel and discipline chronic offenders.

Good Leadership: The Proactive Approach

Achieving acceptable levels of departmental attendance requires leadership skills, especially when working conditions are less than ideal. Supervisors must also screen out job candidates whose history portends attendance problems. Leaders who keep absenteeism under control make special efforts to place employees in jobs that suit their personal interests and work styles. They strengthen the stress resistance of their people while minimizing the amount of stress that they themselves produce (see chapter 4 for more on stress).

Interpret, Promulgate, and Enforce Policies

Policies and rules are ineffective if they are not communicated. It is not enough to enunciate them during orientation programs. Articulate them periodically at staff meetings. Supplement these discussions with facts and figures on the costs of absenteeism and how those individuals who have good attendance records feel about the no-shows.

Remind employees that sick leave represents insurance, not another time-off benefit. Emphasize the point that using up sick leave by taking 1-day absences can leave people in the bind should they need these for lengthy serious illnesses. Emphasize that good attendance is a condition of employment and that attendance records are stored in their personnel files.

Keep attendance records. These should show the number of days absent, the excuses given, and the relationship of these days to holidays, vacations, hunting seasons, and paydays.

Enforce the policies equitably. Do not make exceptions, including yourself and your high performers. Consistency is essential. Do not ignore abuses when things are running smoothly, then crack down when you are short-handed or short-tempered. Do not pick on your poor performers or people you dislike.

Model what you expect from others. People are impressed more by what they see than by what they are told. If the supervisor hobbles to work with a walking leg cast, that provides a good example for her subordinates. If the supervisor comes on board coughing and sneezing, that is a bad model.

Encourage discussions prior to, rather than after, absences. Employees quickly learn that it is easier to ask forgiveness than it is to ask permission.

Insist that people who call in sick talk directly to you. Question them in a supportive manner about their illness. Ask if you can help, how long they think they will be out, and say that they will be missed. When the person is a chronic no-show, do not say, "Gee, I'm sorry. You take whatever time you need to get better." They need to be told to return as soon as possible, or they will take the extra time. Do say (without overdoing the empathy), "Get well fast; we need you here."

At the end of each day, call the employees at home to find out how they are feeling and when you can expect them back. Three benefits are derived from these calls. First, you find out if the person is really at home. Second, it shows that you care about the employee and value her service. Third, when the employee becomes aware of this procedure, she is a little more reluctant to abuse the privilege in the future.

When sick employees return to work, welcome them back and say that they were missed. Inquire as to their problem if you do not already know. Listen carefully if they seem highly stressed and need someone with whom to talk. Even show concern for the chronic abuser of sick leave. Do not react emotionally, nag, or use sarcasm. These are ineffective negative reinforces. Use rational, nonemotional statements such as, "Pat, you have missed two Mondays this month. You are one of our best workers when you are here. What can we do to help?"

Being considerate does not mean being gullible. Do not accept wishy-washy remarks like, "I just did not feel well," or "It was my allergy acting up again." Probe more deeply. Ask how this episode differed from the previous ones, what they did about it, and if the problem is getting better or worse. Watch for verbal or body language signs of uneasiness during this questioning. The phonies become uneasy when these probing discussions continue.

Change the reward/risk ratio. Chronic absenteeism flourishes when the rewards, such as time off to take care of household chores, are greater than the risks involved, such as disciplinary action. This may be on a conscious or a subconscious level. Your goal is to reduce the reward, increase the risk, or both.

Saving unpleasant parts of the chronically absent worker's job for her return or assigning some favorite tasks to others while she is away can reduce the reward. The risk part of the ratio is increased when the absent worker is aware that you notice each of the absences and talk to the employee about each one. This is reinforced when you comment at staff meetings that attendance is a factor in performance appraisals. When people's jobs are in jeopardy, the risk factor escalates.

Counsel and Discipline Chronic Offenders

Even the best-run organizations and departments have a few employees who abuse sick leave, thus necessitating remedial or disciplinary actions. Each attendance problem is unique in some respect. Certainly the variety of excuses offered are endless, so your corresponding solution must be unique for each problem.

Suspect alcohol or drug problems and be on the lookout for evidence of this during work hours. Your primary objective is to alleviate the situation without having to take disciplinary measures. Prepare the groundwork for remedial counseling by acting on the following:

1. Study the employee's attendance record. Note the pattern as well as the number of no-shows, and review the reasons given by the employee. Repetitive patterns usually emerge. To avoid charges of discrimination, review the records of your other workers as well.

2. Review your attendance policy. Because chronic absenteeism is so important and so common, most organizations have documented guidelines for managers. Check these before you take action. Be careful about making threats when the employee has not yet exceeded the number of sick days permitted.

3. If you suspect a drug or alcohol problem, rehearse the exact words you will use to persuade the person to seek professional help.

A precipitating factor always precedes counseling or disciplining actions. For example:

Pat's attendance record is in shambles. Monday, when you arrive at work, you find a message from Pat. She cannot make it in today. You look at all the work left over from the weekend and hear the usual grumbles from Pat's coworkers: "Pat knew that this was inventory day." You have had several brief counseling sessions with Pat, who never seems very concerned, and each time says that she will try harder. Improvement never lasts more than a few weeks. Knowing that supervisors should always have postabsence interviews, you tried to talk to Pat each time she returned from a 1-day absence. She always had a different excuse.

First thing Tuesday morning, you call Pat into your office. This time, you ask your boss if she has time to sit in on the session to emphasize to Pat that you mean business. At the meeting, you remind Pat that everyone would like long weekends, but you realize that this statement has little effect.

Most chronic offenders do not have any feelings of guilt about this. However, you do show Pat that you are on to her little game for getting an extra weekend day.

You pull out Pat's attendance record and hand it to her. The Monday and Friday no-shows have been circled in red by you. You do not ask for more cooperation; you deliver an ultimatum: "One more unexcused absence, and we will be talking about suspensions, Pat." Your boss nods in agreement and makes a little speech about how absenteeism affects the work and the other employees. Pat leaves a lot more impressed than at the end of previous sessions.

As with any chronic problem, this situation has to be monitored closely and any relapse viewed with alarm. Relapsing into old patterns takes place very often. As I said before, absenteeism is not a simple matter.

REFERENCES

1. Greene R. Money for nothing. *Forbes*. 1988;141:48.
2. Morgan PI, Baker HK. Do you need an absenteeism control program? *Supervis Manage*. 1984;29:33-38.
3. Steers RM, Rhodes SR. Major influences on attendance: a process model. *J Appl Psychol*. 1978;63:391-407.
4. Dow S, Markman S. Absenteeism control methods: a survey of practice and results. *Personnel Admin*. 1982;27:73-84.
5. Garreau J. Article in the *Washington Post*. Cited in: *Lancaster Sunday News*, March 14, 1993.
6. Kuzmits FE. No fault: a new strategy for absenteeism control. *Personnel J*. 1981;60:387-390.

19. People Who Resist Change and Avoid Risk

Supervisors in the health care industry have always had to deal with new technology and services, and the rate of these changes continues to escalate exponentially. Fiscal and institutional issues inject additional and more threatening alterations. These developments include the transfer of work from hospitals to other facilities, mergers, acquisitions, new competitors, and complex collaborative efforts.[1] Change does not always represent progress, but progress cannot occur without change.

TYPICAL CHANGES IN HEALTH CARE INSTITUTIONS[2]

- Reorganization
- New leadership
- Restructured jobs
- Changes in methods or procedures
- New equipment, workflow patterns, or technology

Adaptability and flexibility are mandated at all hierarchical levels of a health care organization. When a major change or restructuring occurs, some employees must be completely "recycled." Thus, health care managers today must be change specialists. They must understand why people resist change, persuade employees to view change as normal, and use the best strategies for introducing innovations.

WHY CHANGE IS RESISTED

A militant union leadership can be very resistant to change.[3] However, the major cause for resistance is fear: fear of loss of jobs, fear of loss of working relationships, and fear of inability to do the new work. But mostly, it is fear of the unknown. This fear of the unknown can be minimized by good communication and by including the people who are affected by the change in the planning and implementation processes.

Employees often respond to fear of change, especially when that change may result in loss of job, in stages similar to those experienced by patients with cancer.

1. Denial: "It will not affect me."
2. Anger: "It is not fair; why me?"
3. Bargaining: "Can't there be an exception in my case?"
4. Depression: "Poor me."
5. Acceptance: "I think I can live with this after all."

The stress of change is greatest when employees have existed in a static environment for years and then are suddenly called on to make a change.

STRATEGIES FOR PREVENTING THE PROBLEMS OF CHANGE

Select People Who Do Not Resist Change

Employment history, reference checks, and employment interviews can reveal a tendency to resist change and an unwillingness to take risks. Such evidence should send up the red flag—do not hire these people.

Communicate

The supervisor's role in communicating change can be summed up in three words: tell, sell, and involve. Find out as much as you can from your superiors, peers, and other sources regarding what changes are contemplated. Ask pointed questions about the purpose of the change and how things and people will be affected. The more you learn, the better prepared you will be to answer the many questions that will come your way.

Most CEOs of hospitals have articulated their visions of the future, restated the institutional philosophy, enunciated values, and hung framed mission statements in the main corridor. Department heads are expected to formulate goals and objectives that are congruent with these statements. Ultimately, most efforts to achieve these goals can be translated into change of some sort—and all change involves some risk, to the organization and its employees.

Supervisors must have their own vision of the future for their unit, and this should be shared by their staff.[4] Their vision and goals should be broad enough to include all of the main thrusts of their toil. Objectives represent activities needed to achieve goals. For example, the goal of providing a more competitive laboratory service will require a number of objectives. These would include expansion of services, price reduction, turnaround time, improved facilities, etc.

Explain the need for change and how it benefits the customers, the organization or department, and the employees. Tell them how they will be affected. Provide the reassuring information we mentioned previously. Listen patiently to their fears and alleviate them. Keep them informed at all stages of the change. If appropriate, use charts to show progress during the implementation.[5]

Employees must perceive the change as having more benefits than liabilities. Make yourself available to answer questions. When you do not have an answer, get it for them. Be honest. Straight talk is essential to your credibility. Never use phrases such as, "You know as much about it as I do," or "No one tells me anything either." Avoid the "hard sell." It rarely generates enthusiasm. At best, it leads to acquiescence; at worst, it encourages sabotage.

If ever there was a good example of how a proactive leadership approach is superior to a reactive one, it is in the handling of change. Ask anyone who has been through the ordeal of introducing a hospital information system (HIS). Proactive managers prepare their employees by pointing out the benefits, getting them involved in the planning process, and listening to their advice and concerns before bringing in the equipment. All will likely report that their computer systems were introduced without major difficulties.

Validate Feelings and Provide Reassurance

Attitudes and behavior are difficult to modify unless people feel validated. If they are emotionally tied to an old way, logic and persuasion will fail.[6] Validate employees' feelings by agreeing or empathizing with them. If you say, "I see your point," or "Others have expressed those same feelings," they no longer have the need to defend their viewpoint and are more willing to accept the change. Validation is reinforced when you indicate that despite their reluctance to accept the change, they are still valued by you and by the organization.

It is still more helpful if workers can be reassured that the change will not threaten jobs, assignments, workload, or staffing relationships. Reassurance is also provided when employees are offered transfers or retraining.

They relax when told that jobs will be eliminated only by attrition. They must also be reassured that the change was not introduced because of poor performance on their part.[5]

Empower Employees

Research has shown that people respond more positively to change if they feel they have some control over what is happening. Empower your employees by telling them precisely what you want them to do and, if necessary, showing them how to do it.[4] This knowledge enables them to remove self-doubts and to increase their confidence. This esteem can be enhanced if you express confidence in their ability to adjust to the change. Continue encouragement as it is needed, providing constructive suggestions and caring guidance along the way.

A successful change provides further empowerment.[7] Give employees opportunities to experiment with new behavior in situations where failure is unlikely or would not be very important.

Encourage change in small ways. Involve associates in the planning process. Ask the people who are closest to the job to come up with specific measures. Follow through on as many of their suggestions as possible. Maximize their participation in implementing changes.

Be Patient

No change should be implemented until everyone knows what to expect and has had a chance to express his concerns. Absorb some of the dissonance by patient listening. Give employees time to get used to new ideas. Cushion the stress by accepting temporary decline in performance. Anticipate and tolerate those intense informal discussions around the coffee pot.

Practice What You Preach

Model the behavior, attitude, and comments that you want from your subordinates. For example, when you get the word about a change, do you refer to it as a challenge, look for its best features, agree that it is necessary, and even exhibit enthusiasm? Or, do you groan, wince, or get angry? Do you say things like, "Gosh, now what?" or "What will they expect of us next?" Be willing to take risks and to accept ownership of unpopular ideas.

Reward Participation and Compliance

Provide recognition, praise, and other rewards for contribution of ideas, help in the planning, and participation in the implementation. Minimize the amount of credit you take for success. Talk about your team—lionize others.

COPING WITH PEOPLE WHO OBSTRUCT CHANGE

The Spectators

Spectators are people who are not affected by a change. They have nothing invested in the outcome, and their detachment gives them permission to criticize without contributing.[8] Spectators may watch sympathetically, observe with ill-concealed amusement, or even heckle the employees who are struggling with the change. When you become aware of this behavior, you must put an immediate stop to any sideline nonsense. One way to put a quick halt to this is by assigning to the kibitzers some less desirable tasks related to the change that they find so amusing.

The Nonparticipants

Nonparticipants, unlike the spectators, are affected by a change. They avoid taking an active role because they: (1) perceive the change as having a high risk; (2) think that they may be treated unfairly; (3) expect to be asked to suffer an undue share of the hardships; and (4) anticipate less than a fair share of the benefits.[3] Unless nonparticipants' attitudes affect their teammates or their cooperation is vital to the implementation process, it is probably best to let them remain on the sideline. If it is essential for them to be involved, you and your associates must do a better job of convincing them of the benefits or the necessity of the change.

The Skeptics

Some skeptics are to be expected. Use your enthusiasm and that generated in others to neutralize their negativism. Use the vision you created to demonstrate how favorable outcomes can result. Try to convert these opponents by giving them responsibility for some of the action. Sharing power with critics is effective in selected instances.[4] For example, Supervisor Jan was getting lots of flak at staff meetings from Jack about her plans to implement a hospital "point-of-care" program. This program was passing from a pilot-study phase to a hospital-wide initiative. Jack recommended that the laboratory try to stonewall the effort because, according to him, the program would fail. Jan insisted that Jack spend several days on the nursing unit where the pilot program was in effect. Jack not only stopped his carping, he became an activist for the new service.

The Resisters

Resistance can take the form of procrastination or purposeful obstruction. If you adopt the preventive measures that have been discussed, you will have a much better chance of converting resisters instead of fighting with them. If conversion fails, they must either be removed from the activities related to the implementation of the change or be eliminated from the work team.

The Bosses Who Resist Change

Managers are also susceptible to change resistance. In addition to the fears already mentioned, a manager may fear the loss of power, the perception that he is an inept leader, or the revelation of lack of expertise that he is supposed to possess.

Resistance by managers may be in response to changes mandated by their superiors or—much more likely—in response to suggestions coming from associates or subordinates. In either instance, you may be able to help your boss by offering to assume some of the responsibility for the project. In fact, such situations offer excellent opportunities for career development. For example:

Department heads of a large nursing home have been told to revise all the position descriptions in their departments in order to comply with the new requirements of the Americans with Disabilities Act (ADA). Ann, one of the department chiefs, was trying unsuccessfully to persuade the human resources department to make these revisions. Dan, Ann's assistant, offered to attend a workshop on this subject and then to help with the revisions.

When you propose a change to your boss, you have a better chance for approval if you outline it thoroughly and show that it has a good chance for success, will benefit the department, and will make your boss look good. Provide valid data without holding back any negative factors. Charts, references, and support from experts all help to convince a hesitant boss.

The Risk Avoiders

The word "risk" sends shock waves up and down health care institutions. After all, a great deal of time and expense is allocated to reducing risk. Such efforts include credentialing, certification, instrument maintenance, preventive medicine, safety policies, infection surveillance, environmental testing, and quality assurance. Risk managers and patient representatives continually try to avert possible medicolegal problems.[9]

The risks addressed here are not those that threaten the well-being of patients or employees. Rather, they are the risks related to daily decision making. Every day, managers and professionals make untold numbers of decisions, each involving some risk. Unwillingness to take risks results in inactivity, delays, frustration, and anger. When faced with a decision, top performers match the reward or benefit of a successful action with the penalty of failure, and then they estimate the odds in favor or against success. Ideally the reward is great; the penalty and risk are minimal.

Risk avoiders resist making decisions without first exploring every nook and cranny for bugs. They are very hesitant about committing themselves to new objectives and plans.[3] Instead of acting, they avoid change, pass the buck, and procrastinate. Typical comments of risk avoiders include:

- "They do not pay me enough to make those decisions."
- "I assumed that someone else had to approve it."
- "I did not think I had the authority."

Why do they avoid risks? Before we lay all the blame on these hesitant people, we must consider some legitimate excuses. These employees: (1) may have been severely chastised in the past for sticking their necks out; (2) may not have received any credit or reward for taking risks; or (3) may have bosses who tend to take credit for successes and blame others for failures.

Following are several ways to encourage people to take risks:

1. Include "willingness to take risks" in the list of necessary qualifications in position descriptions.
2. Emphasize innovativeness and resourcefulness when orienting new employees.
3. Teach the skills of decision making.
4. Show employees how to avoid foolish risks and refuse to tolerate repeats of the same errors.
5. Provide the information needed to make intelligent decisions.
6. Ensure early and quick successes at the beginning. Early success encourages risk taking. Reluctant risk-takers need to taste success.
7. Teach them which actions are reversible and which are not.
8. Give them some leeway to be wrong and to realize that some mistakes are part of the price that must be paid for personal and organizational growth and progress.

9. Place minimal restrictions on delegated authority.
10. Do get upset and say so to employees when you hear them tell clients, "I cannot do anything about that," or "I will have to check with my supervisor."
11. Show them that you take risks. A good risk-taker inspires others to do likewise. Talk openly about the errors you have made.
12. Reward risk taking, not risk avoidance.
13. When people goof, do not punish them. Let them criticize their work before you do. This encourages them to look at action from a variety of angles and it sharpens their risk-taking skills for the next time.

REFERENCES

1. Umiker W. *Management Skills for the New Health Care Supervisor.* Rockville, Md: Aspen Publishers; 1988.
2. McConnell CR. *The Effective Health Care Supervisor.* 2nd ed. Rockville, Md: Aspen Publishers; 1988.
3. Giegold WC. *Practical Management Skills for Engineers and Scientists.* Belmont, Calif: Lifetime Learning Publishers; 1982.
4. Belasco JA. *Teaching the Elephant to Dance.* New York, NY: Crown Publishers; 1990.
5. Weiss WH. *The Supervisor's Problem Solver.* New York, NY: AMACOM; 1982.
6. Werther WB Jr. *Dear Boss.* New York, NY: Meadowbrook Press; 1989.
7. Trager MJ, Willard S. *Transforming Stress into Power.* Chicago, Ill: Great Performance Inc; 1988.
8. Gilbreath RD. The myths about winning over resisters to change. *Supervis Manage.* 1990;35:1-3.
9. Umiker W. Risk taking: a supervisory imperative. *MLO.* 1991;23:68-70.

20.   Unethical People

For you to be good is noble. To tell others to be good is even nobler and much less trouble."[1]

Ethics represents what we should do, not necessarily what we must do. It expresses our conscience or morality rather than our acquiescence to legal decrees.[2] It is important to distinguish between ethical and legal behavior. Most illegal actions are also unethical, but there are exceptions (eg, illegal parking is seldom regarded as unethical). Many unethical actions are perfectly legal, which is one reason they are so common.

Unfortunately, everyone does not agree as to what is ethical and what is unethical. Little discordance exists with regard to flagrant violations, but views become murky with less flagrant activities. For example, most observers would regard the theft of a patient's purse as dishonest and unethical, but how about taking home a few office supplies, using the hospital copier for personal papers, or balancing one's checkbook while on duty? Most of us regard repeated abuses of sick leave as unethical, but how about the parent who calls in sick in order to stay home to take care of an ill child?

The daily behavior, decisions, and actions of supervisors are affected by ethics. In any given situation, what a supervisor perceives as "right" affects not only her actions, but also the behavior and attitudes of the people who report to her.[3]

Problems also occur when the ethics of an institution are not congruent with those of its employees. Differences in awareness and interpretation of ethical standards create many dilemmas. This interpretive dissonance is often related to choice of perspective.

THE TWO ETHICAL PERSPECTIVES

1. According to utilitarianism or the consequential perspective, acts are either right or wrong depending on their consequences. In other words, the ends may justify the means. Even outright lies might be justified if they produce more satisfaction than any other method.[4] For instance, a physician who tells a dying patient that recovery is possible justifies that fabrication from a utilitarian perspective. The physician considers the ethical principle of beneficence (the duty to help others) to override the principle of veracity (the duty to be truthful).

2. The "respect for persons" perspective holds that one must refrain from acts that are inherently disrespectful of people—ourselves and others. This view holds that the duty to avoid doing wrong is stronger than the duty to promote good. For instance, the first rule of medical ethics is primum non nocere—first, do not harm. This perspective forbids breach of promise or any other violation of the "golden rule." Lying, manipulative overstatement, or omission are all forbidden.[4] Not informing a new hire that the position is only temporary would be regarded as morally wrong. Telling a patient that she is being given a placebo when she asks would be required.

MEDICAL AND NONMEDICAL ISSUES

Medical issues involve patients—their rights and the decisions or policies that pertain to those rights. These include the right of patients to refuse treatment, the decision to resuscitate or not to resuscitate, and the policy of transferring indigent patients to other facilities. Confidentiality of personal information and medical reports is a sensitive and sometimes complicated issue. For example, who, in addition to the attending physician, may have access to this information? What data may be reported over the phone or via a computer and to whom?

Nonmedical issues include unkept promises, manipulative statements, resident physicians' right to reasonable work schedules, an employer's right to fire a "moonlighting" employee, and accepting gifts in return for preferential treatment.

ETHICS AND THE INSTITUTION

Ethical considerations have received much attention recently; more so because of the threat of legal liability than by strong concern for people.

Organizations are busy formulating and promulgating mission statements. Are these organizations trying to provide meaningful guidelines for ethical behavior, or are they merely articulating public relations messages?[1]

Mission Statements

Lofty mission statements may initially convince employees that loyalty should be to the consumer. Actual practice, however, reflects a different picture when these same employees are instructed to discontinue home care for a patient whose health insurance benefits have expired.[5]

Unequal rights is another danger. The same organization that disciplines a nursing aide for coming to work late may ignore a high-revenue–generating surgeon who reeks of alcohol.[5]

At the other end of the spectrum, we have the exemplary performance by the Johnson & Johnson Company during the highly publicized Tylenol® crisis in which seven people died. Johnson & Johnson promptly ordered every package of that item off the shelves nationwide, even though the deaths were limited to a single city.

A mission statement must convey a commitment of ethical practice. A critical first step is recognition of the fundamental role of values. These corporate values deal with honesty, integrity, loyalty, communication, and customer service. A moral organizational culture is built on value systems.[6] For example:

"The outpatient department is committed to providing high-quality, low-cost, caring service to all patients, without regard for their economic or social status. Our personnel participate actively in the institution's continuing education programs, which feature prompt, high-quality service and high ethical standards."

Policies and Guidelines

Mission statements alone are not enough. They must be backed up with policies and other guidelines that spell out ethical practices. Two examples are patient autonomy and conflict of interest.

All too often patients are handed consent forms to sign without knowing what their choices are or even what they are signing. Institutions must take measures to ensure that options are explained so that patients can make intelligent choices.

Institutions should also develop conflict of interest statements. A conflict of interest exists when a board member or an executive (or a relative) has a financial interest that could be affected by these officers' decisions. Conflict of interest also pertains to "moonlighting" employees who also may have conflicts of loyalty.[7]

Consultative Resources

To assist in facing ethical dilemmas and formulating guidelines, administrators rely on ethics committees, ethics rounds, patient advocacy, and in-service education.[1] Quality assurance committees and ethical review boards also address the moral nature of specific issues.

In this chapter we do not address major biomedical problems such as euthanasia, abortion, organ transplantation, resuscitation decisions, or limiting expensive diagnostic and therapeutic procedures to those that are reimbursable. Instead, we will focus on day-to-day situations that challenge health care supervisors and their colleagues.

ETHICS AND THE SUPERVISOR

Many new forces impacting health care management have added ethical dilemmas. As authority and responsibility shift down the organizational hierarchy, supervisors are increasingly involved in ethical professional and institutional decisions.[5]

Personal vs Organizational Values

Supervisors and professionals have their own beliefs, attitudes, and values about how people should be treated. At times, these personal values conflict with those of the organization (eg, a supervisor who advocates racial equality is given the subtle message that outpatients at that agency prefer white caregivers).[5] Problems such as this are likely to increase as our work force becomes ever more multicultural. Such issues are settled best by open discussion at staff meetings. Reference sources will be discussed later in this chapter.

Selection of Ethical Employers

Ideally, job seekers should consider the ethical environment of an institution when looking for employment.[7] They should inquire about how the organization has dealt with issues that frequently present ethical problems, such as caring for the medically indigent, dealing with neighbors (eg, on-street parking), or the practice of promoting from within.

Supervisory Relationships

Sensitive supervisors consider the impact of their handling of ethical decisions and actions on their superiors, subordinates, and customers (patients, physicians, families of patients, third-party payers, suppliers, and various institutional departments). A strong connection exists between ethical issues and the level of stress experienced by subordinates.[2]

Supervisors must set the ethical tone of the work setting, largely by modeling ethical behavior. If a supervisor is perceived as being unethical, then employees are likely to feel that similar behavior on their part is perfectly acceptable.[3]

Although they might not use the word "ethical," a disturbing number of employees question the integrity or honesty of their leaders. Some recite a litany of broken promises. They note how closely their managers adhere to stated values, especially during a crisis. All too often they witness a sudden shift in the relative importance of quality when services get behind schedule.

Supervisors should see the unfurled flag of ethics when they hear employee statements that include "unfair," "bad," "should," "double-talk," "wrong," or "responsibility."

Following are examples of ethical misadventures by managers:

- When her departmental budget was slashed, the department chief discontinued an important but profit-losing Medicaid service rather than cutting back an inflated departmental roster.
- On Friday afternoon, Diana, a head nurse, gave an inspirational speech on the importance of patient satisfaction. On the following Monday, she took the afternoon off to go shopping, leaving her floor understaffed.
- Phlebotomists attend an in-house seminar on compassionate care giving. Subsequently they spend more time talking with patients during their blood collection rounds. This practice incurs the wrath of their supervisor when they deliver the specimens to the laboratory later than usual.
- Supervisor Dan demonstrates favoritism when approving requests to attend professional meetings.
- Supervisor Jim deprives his boss of honest feedback about how the employees are reacting to a new directive.
- Supervisor Denise waits until the next formal performance appraisal to tell a subordinate what she really thinks of that employee's work.

ETHICAL ISSUES CONCERNING PATIENT CARE

Ethical issues concerning patient care are the most troubling issues faced by care providers. These issues are largely potential violations of patients' rights.[8] Some examples include:

- Confidentiality of records.
- Right to privacy.
- Right to information regarding diagnostic and therapeutic procedures.
- Right to refuse treatment.
- Freedom from harm (eg, discontinuing research project when control patients are getting worse or treated ones experience severe side-effects).

Patients and third-party payers have the right to fair and reasonable charges. Examples of overcharging include:

- Unnecessary diagnostic testing.
- Deliberate double-billing.
- Charging for tests that are part of a research project and would not otherwise have been ordered.
- Billing deceased patients for diagnostic procedures not reported until after the patient had died.

UNETHICAL BEHAVIOR OF SUBORDINATES

Staff members may demonstrate unethical behavior that represents disloyalty to superiors or employers. Unethical staffers may purposely create crises or promote disharmony. Technical specialists sometimes make unreasonable demands, knowing that they are indispensable.

The pilfering of supplies comes under the rubric of theft and is therefore subject to severe penalties. More controversial, and within the realm of ethics, is the "borrowing" of equipment for personal use. Discrimination is often displayed in such situations. For example, a surgeon, without permission, removes an expensive surgical instrument from the surgical suite and uses it at another facility. He brings it back broken, and no one says a word. That same week, a maintenance worker is severely reprimanded when he returns a borrowed power tool.

UNETHICAL BEHAVIOR OF SUPERIORS

Superiors, especially insecure or incompetent ones, often grab credit for ideas generated by their staffers. If they feel that an associate is gaining popularity or power, they may try to impede that person's progress. Some examples of unethical behavior of superiors follow:

- A CEO's son is admitted because of an unsuccessful suicide attempt. The CEO insists on a false medical diagnosis.
- An executive practices subtle exclusion against a junior rival by diverting important information, excluding her from important meetings, and encouraging top management to eliminate her job.
- A pathologist who profits from laboratory work and who is a member of the utilization committee defends staff physicians who overuse laboratory services.
- A technical director falsifies data while preparing for a state inspection.

UNETHICAL BEHAVIOR OF COLLEAGUES

Employees can create dilemmas for their associates who are aware of unethical behavior on the part of these employees. Unfortunately, "whistleblowing," the disclosure of misconduct on the part of others, is often more hazardous to the whistleblower than it is to the offender. For example:

- An emergency room attendant witnesses a physician physically abusing an unruly child.
- In the hospital dining room, a caregiver overhears a colleague naming a patient who has AIDS.
- A nurse observes an anesthesiologist injecting himself with a drug.
- A sales representative falsifies her expense account.
- A laboratory report is not on a patient's chart because the nurse forgot to enter the request into the computer. When the attending physician complains about the missing report, the nurse blames the laboratory.

HOW TO COPE WITH ETHICAL PROBLEMS

To ignore ethical dilemmas or avoid managerial responsibility serves the employer poorly. It is far more useful to recognize and confront ethical dilemmas directly.[5] However, supervisors may want to do what is right but lack the support or information that would permit this.

Education is Essential

Employees are most impressionable when they are first hired. Institutional orientation programs must emphasize the values that reflect the philosophy of the organization. Departmental indoctrination should reinforce this by word and by behavior modeling.

Keep ethos in mind whenever operational or personnel decisions are under consideration. Hold periodic staff meetings to discuss ethical policies and guidelines. Case studies sensitize staff to concerns such as confidentiality, the patient's right to autonomy, and issues of age, race, and gender discrimination.[8]

Dealing With Unethical Superiors

Supervisors may come face to face with situations in which the actions of senior managers are so unethical that the supervisors feel compelled to do something. Options include direct confrontation or reporting the situation to higher authorities (eg, the CEO or the Board of Directors), to a regulatory agency (eg, Equal Employment Opportunities Commission [EEOC] or the Occupational Safety and Health Administration [OSHA]), or to the press. Because disclosures to outside agencies breach the confidentiality and trust that the organization has placed in the protester, this course of action is best limited to major violations.

Even when complaints are perfectly valid and appropriate, the person who blows the whistle is usually viewed as a "snitch." Sometimes the best action is to resign. This move also makes it easier to report the ethical or illegal actions to the proper authorities.

Dealing With Dishonest or Unethical Subordinates

If you are the responsible supervisor, gather solid proof of the unethical activities or behavior of a subordinate; do not rely on rumor or the word of an associate. Document all facts carefully and completely, consult with your superior, and then confront the employee. In many instances, your boss should participate in the confrontation.

Dealing With Dishonest or Unethical Colleagues

Usually, it is best to confront the unethical colleague and tell her that you are aware of what is going on and will have to report it if these transgressions continue. In other situations, that report should be made without an antecedent warning. Judgment is required in so many ethical dilemmas.

Reference Sources

Institutional ethics committees address policy issues and advise personnel on specific ethical concerns and dilemmas. However, these committees are most often concerned with issues of patient care rather than relationships between employees or between employees and supervisors. Committees that address quality assurance, utilization review, and medical audits often find themselves struggling with ethical concerns.[8] Many professionals and supervisors are members of organizations, such as the American Medical Association, that publish formal codes of ethics to guide their members on professional behavior. Such ethical codes may be too broad for daily use.[8] When specific problems arise, seek assistance from other members of the management team in resolving differences between personal beliefs and the activities of the organization.[7] Religious leaders are always able and willing to advise.

REFERENCES

1. Storch JL. Teaching ethics: preparing health services managers for ethical decision making. *J Health Admin Ed.* 1988;6:287-297.
2. Bissell M, Cosman T. How ethical dilemmas induce stress, part 1. *MLO.* 1991;23:28-33.
3. Rue LW, Byars LL. *Supervision: Key Link to Productivity.* Homewood, Ill: Richard D. Irwin; 1982.
4. Dougherty CI, Cederblom J. The right choice: two approaches to determining right and wrong. *Health Prog.* 1990;71:86-89.
5. Eliopoulos C. Ethics and the health care supervisor. *Health Care Supervis.* 1988;6:27-37.
6. Rindler M. *Putting Patients and Profits Into Perspective.* Chicago, Ill: Pluribus Press; 1987.
7. Gould GR, Younkins EW. Guidelines help managers deal with ethical issues. *Healthcare Fin Manage.* 1989;43:32-36.
8. Anderson GR, Glesnes-Anderson VA. Ethical thinking and decision making for health care supervisors. *Health Care Supervis.* 1987;5:1-12.

21. Bad Attitudes and Pessimists

The employees who give supervisors their biggest headaches are not the incompetent ones—they can be trained. They are not the ones who brazenly violate rules—they can be disciplined. Rather, they are the subordinates who meet work standards but who drive supervisors up the wall with their bad or negative attitudes.

Mellott[1] says that these people have an effect on you like swallowing steel marbles: "By the end of the day you feel weighted down and tired. You may regurgitate the pellets, pelting the culprit or some innocent bystander."

BAD ATTITUDE IS NOT THE ONLY CAUSE OF BAD BEHAVIOR

This brings up an old polemic: "What comes first, attitude or behavior?" While supervisors are correct when they attribute poor performance to poor attitude, studies and empirical observations have demonstrated that attitudes change as the result of behavior modifications. The U.S. Marine Corps learned this generations ago. Marine instructors will tell you that they do not care what a recruit's "attitude" is when he joins. By the time recruits complete their basic training, most of them have developed pride in themselves and their organization. Attitudinal problems disappear as a result of behavior modification. The reason for this transformation is complex, but skill enhancement and pride in one's unit are undoubtedly significant factors.

When confronted with employees who are misbehaving or underperforming, supervisors often jump to the conclusion that bad attitudes are at the root of the problems. While bad attitudes usually *do* result in behavioral variances, most behavioral variances are *not* caused by bad attitudes. The many other and more common causes include unclear supervisory expectations, lack of orientation and training, peer influence, lack of congruence between employee and job, monotonous tasks, faulty communication, or feedback systems that punish good performance and reward poor performance. Bad attitude should be the last, not the first, etiology to be considered when diagnosing behavior problems.

Additionally, since we cannot get into our employees' heads, our diagnosis of "bad attitude" is based on a very tenuous assumption. For this reason, we should never accuse an employee of having a bad attitude or, for that matter, of having a poor work ethic, being unprofessional, or lacking motivation. These are all judgmental, subjective accusations. Instead, we should articulate what we see or hear—behavior or dialogue—and this demands objectivity and specificity. For example, instead of, "The trouble with you is that you have a bad attitude," say, "I have heard you make disparaging remarks about our unit, your attendance has plummeted during the past three months, and the night shift is complaining that you leave work for them to finish up." With that said, let's move on to the people with bad attitudes.

A person with a bad attitude may be a negativist, a goof-off, a hothead, a disciplinary problem, or a disloyal subordinate. The two common denominators of employees with bad attitudes are thinly veiled or open antagonism toward supervisors and an unhealthy reaction toward their job, the workplace, or the people in it. To alter the underlying attitudes is difficult; to alter the resulting behavior is less difficult. More importantly, behavior modification can impact attitude adjustment.

Negative individuals are too clever to be openly insubordinate; their defiance is more subtle. They demonstrate a proclivity for ignoring requests and often become disruptive centers of bickering. Your requests are met with, "You cannot be serious," "They do not pay me enough to do that," or "What is in it for me?"

Rarely do they volunteer for anything, and they can find a million-and-one reasons for not doing what they do not want to do, especially when it comes to activities such as working weekends or overtime. When you look to delegate to someone, you never give these folks a second thought. You would gladly trade in one of these difficult people for a pair of used rubber gloves.

Negative attitudes may be reflected in low productivity, high error rate, violation of rules and procedures, lack of team spirit, uncooperativeness, public criticism of the organization and its officers, or constant threats to resign—just about any undesired behavior. It is often difficult to draw the line between bad attitude and disloyalty or bad attitude and unethical behavior. For example:

Gert challenges as many policies as she can without overstepping the line. She comes to work on time, then rushes off to the cafeteria for a leisurely breakfast. Her personal appearance leaves much to be desired, but she does not quite violate the dress code. She rarely makes positive comments at staff meetings; she often just sits there and glowers. At performance reviews, you find yourself spending most of the time arguing over Gert's ratings. She shows no interest in accepting more responsibility or formulating career improvement plans. Her favorite remark is, "Let's skip all that rhetoric and talk about my salary."

Percy is another classic example of someone with an attitudinal problem. He thinks he should have your job. He is sullen, cranky, complaining, and hypercritical. He has been overheard in the coffee shop bad mouthing you and the organization.[2] Percy tips off his attitude with, "You should not ask me to do that. It is not in my position description." There are three effective responses to that cop-out: (1) add that task to the job description; (2) maintain that the task is included under the umbrella statement "other duties as assigned"; or (3) regard such responses as indicative of poor cooperation, something that will be reflected in the next performance rating.

If supervisors had the courage to document what they really thought about their Gerts and their Percys, the following adjectives would appear in their performance appraisal reports: disinterested, inflexible, pessimistic, complaining, indifferent, change resistant, unenthusiastic, and unsupportive.

WHY DO THEY HAVE BAD ATTITUDES?

The etiology of bad attitudes is complex and multifactorial in most instances and varies from person to person. Behavioral psychologists report two frequent factors: low self-esteem and a need for attention. A difference of "chemistry" between employee and supervisor is frequently mentioned, but other more substantive causes are usually at play. Some of the most pernicious forms originate in early childhood—the "gift" of a negative life script from parents.

Poor outlooks may be brought to a new job from elsewhere or may be developed on the job. Boredom, distasteful tasks, low salary, unpleasant work environment, and incompatible associates may serve as causes or aggravating factors. Employees who are overqualified—or who think they are—often have less than adequate attitudes.

A major reason why these employees continue to act as they do is that the reward/risk ratio of this negative behavior is high. The rewards include escape from extra or unpleasant work, getting attention (negative strokes are better than no strokes), and the perverse pleasure of tormenting a disliked superior. Undesired behavior will decrease if you can lower the ratio by decreasing the reward and/or increasing the risk. For instance, the reward can be reduced by shunning the person when they function in their negative mode. The risk can be increased by assigning them less pleasant tasks despite their loud protests.

THAT OLD SELF-FULFILLING PROPHECY

Frustration and anger lead supervisors to distance themselves from negative people, but this only aggravates the employee's low self-esteem. Gert feels neglected and ostracized. This activates a self-fulfilling prophecy. The negative expectations on the part of the boss impacts unfavorably on Gert's subsequent behavior, and she then performs according to these low expectations.

HOW TO COPE WITH INDIVIDUALS WITH BAD ATTITUDES

The quality of supervision has a major impact on employee attitude. Attitude varies directly with morale and motivation. Good supervision can lead to significant and widespread attitudinal improvement. Workers who see their jobs as a positive part of their life because their boss is sincere and sees the good in their performance are more satisfied with their work and do a better job. Under the leadership of a new supervisor, a disgruntled employee may exhibit a remarkable conversion.

The Generic Approach

Before taking any action with an employee, determine if a problem really exists. In previous chapters we posed the critical question that comes up whenever we face a difficult person. It is worth repeating: Does the behavior affect to a significant degree the department's work, the difficult person's coworkers, or you? If not—and you think you can learn to live with it—your best move may be no move.

If coaching alone does not get the desired change, move on to counseling. Discuss the problem with the person candidly. Explain how the behavior affects you, the department, or others. Give specific examples of how you see the person's disenchantment being expressed and how it affects you.[2]

Talk About Behavior, Not Attitude

When we tell people that they have a poor attitude, we must be able to provide specific behavioral examples that led to that subjective diagnosis. Failing to do that, whether in a performance review or a counseling session, we will: (1) elicit defensiveness or anger; (2) confuse our subject; and (3) not get the desired behavioral change.

When we get into that trap, we find ourselves in a "No I don't"/"Yes you do" argument that gets us nowhere. Even if the person agrees (eg, "I guess

you must be right, my wife tells me the same thing"), he has only
ideas for altering that attitude. We must focus on specific offending ᴮᴱᴴ
ior. Here is an example of how a skillful office manager translated attitude
into behavior:

> Doctor: "That new receptionist has a bad attitude."
> Office Manager: "What makes you say that, Doctor?"
> Doctor: "He does not treat us with respect."
> Office Manager: "What does he do or not do to make you say that?"
> Doctor: "Well, for one thing, he calls me by my first name."
> Office Manager: "Anything else?"
> Doctor: "When he cannot find a report and I complain about the lousy
> service, he shrugs his shoulders and says, 'I only work here.'"
> Office Manager: "Anything else?"
> Doctor: "That should be enough—I have got to run."
> (later) Office Manager to receptionist: "Please call physicians by their
> formal name, Glen. And, when you cannot find a report right away,
> do not shrug your shoulders and say something like, 'I only work
> here.' That turns our clients off."

Likewise, instead of saying, "You have a bad attitude," use "I" language
and describe what it is that annoys you (eg, "Larry, when I make a legitimate
request, I do not want to hear a lot of grumbling and pouting. It really
upsets me"). This statement has three advantages: (1) it focuses on specific
behavior rather than attitude; (2) it attacks that behavior and not the person; and (3) it lets the person know how you feel about it.

Coaching should be documented. Detailed record keeping should begin
when the results of coaching and counseling are not effective. Cutting these
folks loose may be the best solution, but you will need concrete proof of how
the bad attitude affected performance or other employees.[2]

EMPLOYEES WHO TAKE ADVANTAGE OF THEIR EMPLOYERS

Employees who take advantage of their employers do only what is absolutely
required. They remain aloof and do not cooperate with their coworkers.
They perform marginally, avoid additional work, and complain loud and
often. They are great for pointing out any deficiencies in the completeness of
your department's position descriptions.

To counteract these hangers-on, you must define their duties and
responsibilities more precisely. At the next performance review or in counseling sessions, describe your expectations, especially how you expect better
cooperation and teamwork. If they are not pulling their share of the load,
give them your best motivational talk on the benefits of team spirit to everyone. Discuss how their reluctance to go the extra mile makes everyone's job

more difficult and affects their performance ratings. Emphasize that everybody has to get their hands dirty once in a while.

Be wary of making accusations of disloyalty. That term, like that of attitude, is too subjective. Stick to what you can see or hear.

Get them more involved in planning and taking ownership of ideas or projects. Praise them for any behavioral change in the right direction. Do not wait until their performance reaches the ultimate behavioral level you would like them to attain before you applaud their achievements.

EMPLOYEES WHO ARE HYPERCRITICAL OF THEIR EMPLOYERS

In most instances, mouthing off by one or two employees is not serious. Often it can be nipped in the bud by a remark such as, "For someone with your ability, I cannot understand why you would stay with this organization. Don't you find it demeaning?"[3]

In two instances, however, you must take vigorous action before serious harm is produced. The first is when these people bad-mouth the organization in front of patients, visitors, clinicians, or other customers. The second is when they advise other employees to slow down. These two situations justify charges of disloyalty, and in most organizations are grounds for dismissal. Give them appropriate warning. Read your organization's policy manual or the employee's handbook or consult with your human resources department. Then take appropriate action.

THE PESSIMISTS

We must differentiate between an employee with a negative attitude and a pessimist, or "wet blanket." The latter is a person who finds fault with everything and everybody. Pessimists may be hard workers who are competent, productive, and even loyal, but they have a bleak outlook toward most things and most people. They lack excitement in life and happiness at work. If you hang around them long enough, you get infected. Soon you are talking like they do. People tend to avoid them, and so would you if it were not for the fact that this pessimist reports to you or works side by side with you.

Pessimists are convinced that those who have power cannot be trusted or counted on to act reasonably and consistently. Because they believe that others in power do not care or are self-serving, their negative statements are made with conviction.[4] In meetings, when any new idea is proposed, pessimists can be counted on to come up with, "The trouble with that idea is...."

Pessimists may be confused with devil's advocates. Both voice concern or ask challenging questions, but the devil's advocate does so with an open mind and is prepared to join a consensus if convinced. The pessimist persists in finding reasons for opposing whatever is being proposed no matter what. When pessimists lose arguments or are outvoted, they remain unconvinced. Nevertheless, do not dismiss their comments too quickly. This could turn the others present against you. Keep your group thinking positively.

General Principles for Dealing With Pessimists

1. Avoid acceptance of the contrary outlooks expressed by these individuals. Their resistive persuasion is not only depressing and self-defeating, it can be infectious.

2. When a known pessimist is present at a meeting, do not rush into making suggestions. Describe the problem thoroughly and call for solutions from others. Pessimists tend to remain silent while a problem is being explored or when alternatives are being solicited. They spring into action after solutions have been proposed.

3. Project realistic optimism. Give examples of past successes of the action now being proposed. Concede that every action carries some element of risk. Point out that failure to take action is riskier than taking the wrong action. Using a worst-case scenario, show that the possible consequences are not threatening, and the chances for success are great. Explain that current conditions are not like those present before when a similar project was not successful. Relate favorable outcomes that other departments or organizations experienced using the same actions.

4. Do not argue—you will not convince them. Your goal is not so much to convert them as it is to get them to be more cooperative and less vocal. It is the other participants whom you want to convince. Avoid arguments by simply stating that the pessimist may be right, but that you want to go on or that you agree with the others on the best course of action.

5. If the pessimists persist, press for details as to why the proposal will not work or insist that they come up with alternatives. Assign them information-gathering chores. Each time the pessimists try to kill a suggestion, demand that they come up with positive alternatives.

6. Have an open mind. Once in a while the pessimists may be right. Use their negativism when you get to discussing pitfalls and contingency planning. They can tell you everything that can go wrong.[4]

7. Be prepared to take appropriate action by yourself, even if the group remains under a pessimist's spell.[4]

8. If the pessimist is a colleague and the work situation does not demand that you work together, avoid him if you value your optimism.

9. Do not encourage negativism. When someone says something negative about another person or department, we tend to nod in agreement and add a critical remark of our own.[5] Instead ask, "What do you think we should do about what you just criticized?" If you make it clear that you expect criticism to lead to action, people will be more selective about what they criticize, and when they do criticize, everyone will expect them to take action.[5]

Suggested verbal responses to pessimists include:

- "Bob, you say that Cheryl's suggestion will not work. What will work?"
- "Jane, what is the worst that can happen if we approve this proposal?"
- "You may be right, Anne, but I still want to try this new procedure."
- "I think that if we assume a more optimistic attitude toward this situation, things are likely to work out better."
- "We must take some risks. Nothing would ever be accomplished if we are immobilized by fear."
- "I respect your experience, Jim, but things have changed since the incident you referred to occurred. Let me continue, and you can say more after I have finished."[6]

REFERENCES

1. Mellott R. *Stress Management for Professionals* [audiotapes]. Boulder, Colo: CareerTrack Publications; 1987.
2. Danziel MM, Schoonover SC. *Changing Ways*. New York, NY: AMACOM; 1988.
3. Weiss WH. *The Supervisor's Problem Solver.* New York, NY: AMACOM; 1982.
4. Bramson RM. *Coping With Difficult People.* New York, NY: Random House; 1981.
5. Werther WB. *Dear Boss.* New York, NY: Meadowbrook Press; 1989.
6. Tucker RK. *Fighting It Out With Difficult People.* Dubuque, Iowa: Kendall Hunt Publishers; 1987.

22.   Complaints and Chronic Complainers

We are all complainers, but most of us are not chronic complainers. Listen to a typical group of employees sitting at a table in the cafeteria or relaxing in the employees' lounge. What you are likely to hear are complaints or criticism, usually directed at the boss or the top brass.

Are all complaints bad? No! None of us like to get them, but they serve us well. Complaints from customers provide opportunities to correct something that we would not otherwise have known about. It is much better to have customers complain about our service and to continue to use it, than for them to not complain and stop using it. In fact, complaints represent a major source of customer feedback—the only source for customer input in many health care institutions. Organizations that strive for service excellence search diligently for negative as well as positive feedback from their clients.

What about employee complaints? Isn't it better to have employees complain than to have them resign, bad-mouth the organization, or engage in sabotage? Legitimate or not, complaints are symptoms that somewhere something is wrong and demands attention.

COMMON CAUSES OF EMPLOYEE COMPLAINTS

1.   Job fits (eg, employees are under- or overqualified).
2.   Policies and rules:
     Unwritten or unclear.

193

Outmoded (eg, old dress code).

Difficult or impossible to comply with (eg, brief meal breaks but long lines in cafeteria).

Offensive or demeaning (time clocks, physician certification of 1-day absences, phone use restrictions).

Unfair or inconsistent enforcement.

3. Working conditions:

Low-comfort environment.

Lack of safety measures.

Interrupted or missed work breaks.

Poor physical layouts.

Equipment breakdown.

Shoddy supplies.

4. Compensation and benefits.

5. Competency of leaders (favoritism or poor staffing).

6. Relationships with other employees (harassing or intimidating coworkers).

The supervisor's role is to respond effectively and promptly to legitimate complaints. This avoids formal and often costly grievances. Increasing numbers of lawsuits are being registered by disgruntled employees who think that they have no other option if they want their complaints addressed. Grievances are most likely to be filed following disciplinary action against the aggrieved employees.

The importance of prompt and satisfactory responses to legitimate complaints cannot be overstated. Such action preserves morale and productivity and reduces errors. It is essential for acceptable quality of work life.

What are the appropriate channels for soliciting suggestions and complaints? Yes, supervisors must solicit complaints, which can be euphemistically referred to as "suggestions for improvement." These are aired at staff meetings, performance reviews, exit interviews, and daily contacts—another benefit of managing-by-wandering-around.

Observant supervisors suspect problems when they note that an employee is unusually silent, irritable, or depressed. Caring managers should engage in "naive listening" when they realize that they have started to tune out people such as long-term patients, loquacious colleagues, or boring bosses. Naive listening is listening as though meeting these people for the first time, without preconceived notions.

THE SIX ESSENTIAL STEPS IN ADDRESSING INDIVIDUAL COMPLAINTS

1. Listen carefully. Remember that the initial complaint is often only a trial balloon to see how you will react. It is not the real com-

plaint, only the tip of an iceberg. You may have to dive deeply to find what is under the surface.

2. Investigate. Is the complaint legitimate? Are there less obvious but more serious ones trailing behind? Are other people affected? Is the situation getting better or worse?

3. Decide on what, if any, action is needed. Get help if you need it. Ask the complainer what she would like done. Make certain that your solution will not make matters worse. For example, Supervisor Louise responded to Sue's complaint about the crowded hospital parking facilities by permitting Sue to come to work earlier. Now, all of Sue's coworkers want the same privilege.

4. Inform the complaining employee about your findings and what you propose to do. Provide this information within 24 hours. If your remedy is not satisfactory, look for alternatives.

5. Implement your decision.

6. Check the effectiveness of your action.

"I WOULD LIKE TO TALK TO YOU ABOUT MY RAISE"

While we are on the subject of employee complaints, a universal favorite of workers is dissatisfaction with pay changes. Gripes are heard every year when salary changes are announced. When competitors give larger raises, or at least that is what the rumor mill reports, trouble brews. Similar situations arise when favoritism is thought to be the reason that one person gets a larger increment than do other members of a work group.

The introduction of pay-for-performance strategies has exacerbated salary dissatisfaction. Employees who do not receive the maximum salary increase are often dissatisfied with their performance rating. Even more unhappy are those who were told that their work had been outstanding, then found a minuscule increase in the size of their paycheck.

Suggestions for Avoiding Salary Controversies

1. Do not overrate employees or make unrealistic promises. This is not easy because inflated ratings are the rule. For example, a study of U.S. Navy officer evaluations found that 98.5% of all officers were judged to be "outstanding" or "excellent." Only 1% were rated "average."[1]

2. Know what your competitors are paying. Organizations that enjoy less employee turnover usually maintain salary levels in the upper 25% of those of their competitors.

3. Know exactly how salary increases are determined in your organization.
4. Circumvent salary ceilings for deserving senior staffers. For example, a change in title or responsibilities may make such an employee eligible for a more substantial salary increase.
5. Let employees blow off steam. Be empathetic.
6. Do not be drawn into comparison debates. Refuse to discuss salaries of other employees.
7. Do not be guilty of favoritism.

Following are suggested responses when dealing with salary complaints:

■ "Sue, here is a copy of our recognition and reward policy. After you have read it, we will go over your salary change."
■ "A recent survey showed that our pay scales are competitive."
■ "Take a look at our new benefits package. It makes the bottom line look a lot different."
■ "While salary increases are based largely on performance, other factors must be considered. These include the supply and demand for certain kinds of employees, budgetary restrictions, and the relative numbers of employees in each performance level."
■ "We are having a real financial crunch this year."
■ "We must remain competitive."
■ "The decision was made to reduce salary increments this year rather than lay people off."

WHAT TO DO WHEN CONFRONTED WITH A GROUP OF COMPLAINERS

Bernstein and Rozen[2] recommend what they call "creative ignoring." Just sit still and look thoughtful. This response gets them to quiet down and become more manageable. If it is a group of customers or colleagues, ask for each person's individual input before responding. Then call on the least hostile person to lead off.

If you are met with a bevy of angry subordinates, ask them to pick one spokesperson because you insist on a one-to-one confrontation. Request that the rest of them leave your office. Another alternative is to tell them that you want to talk to each one, but one at a time.

CHRONIC COMPLAINERS

We all have our share of gripes, justified or not. Some of us have rather low thresholds of dissatisfaction, so we complain more than others. The legitimate complainer differs from the chronic complainer in four ways: (1) chronic complainers' complaints are less likely to be valid; (2) chronic complainers are more interested in registering feelings than in getting problems resolved; (3) chronic complainers are seldom willing to participate in finding or implementing solutions; and (4) the daily conversation of chronic complainers consists predominantly of complaints or negative comments.

The occasional gripers can often be stopped in their tracks with, "Well, what are YOU going to do about that," but this does not stop certified chronic complainers. They have had that fired at them too often. They merely throw the ball back into your lap by telling you that they have no influence in the organization or that their suggestions are never taken seriously.

Whiners are simply chronic complainers who add a plaintive vocal register to their complaining repertoire. Whiners sound just like youngsters in the supermarket who want to go home. You hear their mothers say, "No, you cannot have one of those—and stop your whining!" Wouldn't you like to issue the same command to the whiners at work? If you work closely with one of these individuals, you can still hear her mournful voice reverberating after you have returned home.

Tell-tale Characteristics of Chronic Complainers

1. Chronic complainers "gunnysack" problems. When the bag is full, they pull out one or two and hand them to you. They rarely have any solutions in their bags.
2. Chronic complainers constantly use certain words like "never" or "always." This provides you with the opportunity to challenge their observations, since there is seldom a "never" or "always" situation. Their favorites include, "They never consider us," and "We always get the dirty end of the stick." They also articulate many "if only's" or "why doesn't someone...?"
3. Their complaining exacerbates when they are faced with new or challenging tasks—they are getting their alibis ready.
4. While chronic complainers' main criticisms are directed at their leaders, their peers and others do not escape their barbs. They also let you know that competitors are much more competent.
5. The work performance of chronic complainers is usually acceptable despite all their griping. The typical chronic complainer is a conscientious and competent worker unless flexibility and risk-taking are required.

Why Are They Always Complaining?

Chronic complainers see an imperfect world and feel powerless to do anything about it. They suffer from a state of constant frustration because of this feeling of powerlessness and because they are convinced that no one else has the ability or interest to rectify imperfect situations.[3]

The objectives of their complaining are: (1) to do what they think is their duty—to bring a problem to the attention of others; (2) to disclaim any responsibility for correcting the situation—complaining makes them feel blameless and morally perfect; (3) to transfer that responsibility to someone else; and (4) to show that their superiors lack competency (if they cannot be stars, they like to shoot down those who might be).

Chronic complainers derive satisfaction from the complaining process itself. Although they will usually complain to anyone who will listen, they frequently unload on people who lack the authority to do anything about the problems. As a result, chronic complainers seldom get action, and the persistence of the problems confirms their feelings of powerlessness.

Coping With Chronic Complainers

While you rarely cure bona fide chronic complainers, you can often achieve the following:

- Their complaining decreases to a tolerable level.
- They learn to bring you only things that you can do something about.
- They bring solutions with the problems.
- They spend more time performing, less time griping.
- They develop more confidence in their own ability.
- They do not complain in front of customers or your boss.
- They redirect their energy toward problem resolution from that of getting affirmation of their feelings.

If you convert a chronic complainer into a troubleshooter or a supportive devil's advocate, give yourself a pat on the back—you have accomplished what most of us have not.

PRACTICAL SUGGESTIONS FOR DEALING WITH COMPLAINERS

You are not going to change complainers, so either accept them for what they are (insecure individuals with low self-esteem) or get rid of them. That decision is based on how valuable they are and the impact their complaining has on you and your team.

How to Listen to Them

Listening attentively is not easy. What you would like to say is, "Not again. Stop your griping and go back to work." However, being heard can lessen their sense of powerlessness.[3] If you fail to pay attention to their complaints, you will not only aggravate the situation, but you may divert the complaining to people who may get a bad impression about your organization (eg, customers or competitors). If their complaining bypasses you to your superiors, your reputation as a leader will not be enhanced.

Listen to their main points. Write the complaint down—it is good for their self-esteem. Sometimes simply listening can quiet the complainer. Do not agree or disagree with them. Avoid approval nods or sympathetic grimaces. Maintain a noncommittal facial expression. Do not pass judgment on the merits of their complaints.

Direct your attention more at their feelings than at the object of their complaints. They are reassured when their feelings are validated (eg, "I can understand why you are upset about that"). Validating feelings is not the same as agreeing with them—it is only acknowledging their right to have those feelings.

Stop them when they start repeating or they try to move to another topic. Do this politely, but firmly. Rein in rambling discussion by asking, "What is your point?" Acknowledge that you understood what they said by paraphrasing and summarizing their main points.

Answer bad with good. Whatever chronic complainers gripe about, bring up a good point instead of agreeing (eg, "You say that..., but it is been our experience that..."). This makes chronic complainers uncomfortable, and they will tend to focus on legitimate complaints that should be addressed.[2]

Do not try to argue them out of their negative stand, placate them, or explain everything. These tactics seldom work. Do a reality check. Ask them what it is they want you to do or what they would like to see happen. Be honest when you say what you can and will do and what you cannot and will not do. When they say that what you propose will not succeed, ask what is the worst that can happen, then indicate that you are not worried about that state of affairs. Another ploy is to narrow the options to two, and ask which they think is the lesser of the two evils.[4]

Democratic management can only go so far.[5] When solutions are beyond your control, say so. Avoid "I" orientation ("I cannot/I will not"), because it implies you have some discretion in the matter. At times you must make statements like, "Everybody has got to compromise; you are not the only one" or "We have simply got to make the best of it."[5]

Get Them to Problem-Solve

After acknowledging that a problem exists, move quickly into problem solving. Ask specific open-ended questions. These are the who, when, where, and how questions. Avoid the why's because they get you into deep water. True chronic complainers are not comfortable with problem-solving questions—they do not want questions or solutions, they just want you to agree with their complaints.

Suggest a course of action to get them to think in terms of solutions (eg, "You are closer to this than I am, Steve; how would you solve this?").

Assign them something to do to solve the problem (eg, prepare a rough draft of a proposal). This may communicate the fact that they do have the power to get things done. Have them seek out more information. Say, "Steve, as you track these down, jot down at least three things that you think will improve the situation." If they say that they do not have the time, respond by saying, "Well, if you change your mind let me know."

Complete the Interaction

Thank them for bringing you the problem, as you escort them toward the door.

THE DOS AND DON'TS OF COPING WITH COMPLAINERS

Do

- Keep them busy. Complaints surface and multiply during slack periods. They diminish when people are busy or have tasks that require concentration.
- Encourage subordinates to bring their problems to you rather than voicing them to others—especially to customers and outsiders.
- Make complainers aware of the negative effect that their comments have on the people around them.
- Tell complainers that they are jeopardizing their own standing by criticizing management or their employer. Point out that public bad-mouthing of the organization is grounds for disciplinary action and will not be tolerated.

Don't

- Agree that the complaints are correct, even if they are. Saying, "You are absolutely right," encourages more complaining.
- Try to placate them or provide detailed explanation. They are immune to these ploys.
- Ignore a chronic complainer's invitation to listen to her gripes.

- Solve their problems for them.
- Accept blame. Confessions seldom achieve anything. Your admission just validates for them the fact that it is your fault and that they are blameless.[3]
- Apologize. They will only complain more.
- Argue with the complainer. Just say where you stand.
- Become defensive or emotional. Listening unemotionally to criticism shows maturity and lets you take advantage of good ideas that defensiveness and denial would obscure.
- Permit complaining in front of patients or other customers.
- Expect rational approaches to work consistently. You may receive no acknowledgment at all or only a new round of complaining.
- Let them bait, harass, or intimidate you.[5]

REFERENCES

1. Koontz H, O'Donnell C. *Management: A Book of Readings*. 4th ed. New York, NY: McGraw-Hill; 1976.

2. Bernstein AJ, Rozen SC. *Dinosaur Brains: Dealing With All Those Impossible People at Work*. New York, NY: John Wiley & Sons; 1989.

3. Bramson RM. *Coping With Difficult People*. New York, NY: Random House; 1981.

4. Quick TL. *Managing People at Work*. New York, NY: Executive Enterprises Publishing; 1983.

5. Straub JT. Dealing with complainers, whiners, and general malcontents. *Supervis Manage*. 1992;34:1-2.

23.   People Who Have Annoying Habits

This chapter describes a potpourri of characters. Each group displays three unifying characteristics: (1) its members irritate or embarrass their superiors or others; (2) disciplinary measures are usually not appropriate; and (3) their overall work results are acceptable. The annoying habits of this group generally involve personality quirks, which are resistant to external modification. Moreover, members of this group are often colleagues, customers, or superiors over whom we have little or no authority. Even when they are people who report to us, their behavior seldom justifies disciplinary measures. Therefore, most supervisors either avoid these people or tolerate their idiosyncrasies. We will present some approaches that can help to cope more effectively with such individuals.

THE KNOW-IT-ALLS

These authorities on everything want you to recognize them as being superior. They try to maintain control by accumulating large bodies of knowledge. They are condescending if they know what they are talking about, pompous if they do not. Their constant intimidation and belittling makes their associates feel incompetent and humiliated. They are atrocious listeners and they brush off all suggestions—responding with irritation, anger, or withdrawal. If you object to what they say, they take it as a personal affront. When things go wrong, they say, "I told you so" or "What do you expect from the incompetents hired by the idiots in personnel."

Solution: Avoid these insufferable people as much as possible. Do not pose a threat or argue. Remain respectful and avoid direct challenges. Do your homework. Do not stick your neck out; be certain that you know what you are talking about. Present your ideas tentatively, using phrases like, "What would happen if..." or "I wonder if...."

To get them to consider alternative views, align yourself with their ideas. For example, after the self-proclaimed expert has outlined a proposal for scheduling outpatient diagnostic procedures, show enthusiastic support for the overall plan, then piggy-back your modifications.

Resist the temptation to debate them. Backtrack and then repeat what they say. That gets them to listen to you because they bask in their own words. Instead of challenging them, ask probing or extensional questions such as a series of, "Then what would you do?" This forces them to take a second look at their concept.[1] State that you still have some reservations and will have to give it more consideration.

If you want to make a point, but are afraid that the KNOW-IT-ALL will humiliate you in front of others, use the strawperson approach described previously (eg, "How would you respond to someone who claims that your report lacks statistical validity?").

At times you must swallow your pride and acknowledge their competence. If the person is your boss, and you are subjected to this torture daily, learn as much as you can from the person and then resign.[1]

THE FAKE KNOW-IT-ALLS

These phonics simulate the first group, but their knowledge is very superficial. They want attention so badly that they deceive others and even themselves as to what they really know. Although they sound convincing, they are easily tripped up by people who know what the score is. They differ from liars in that they really believe what they say.

These windbags make the most of the bits of knowledge they pick up. They are adept at scanning reports and other published materials. In conversations, it is surprising how many tidbits they accumulate when at the same time they always seem to be doing all of the talking.

Because of their pomposity, it is tempting to shoot them down when you catch them in over their heads—but do not do it! They have a major self-esteem problem, and therefore their behavior demands more compassionate treatment. Your goal is to counter their misinformation or distortions without putting them on the defensive.[2]

Solution: To determine their knowledge on a topic, ask for specifics. Let them down gently by presenting your data as an alternative set of facts. Even better, congratulate them on what they said and then merge your ideas into theirs. In some cases, it is best to say nothing but to get them aside later and clue them in on the real facts. Praise them when their messages are more factual, to reinforce what you want.[2]

THE UNCOOPERATIVE SILENT ONES

These people are not those who do not speak up because they have nothing to say or are listening intently. They are not the polite ones who fear that they will say something wrong or will hurt your feelings. The UNCOOPER-ATIVE SILENT ONES are those who exude fear or suppressed anger by their silence.

Their silence may be preceded by a perfectly congenial conversation until you suddenly touch on a sensitive area. You are most likely to encounter this glum silence during a counseling or disciplinary session. For example:

You have just greeted Irene, one of your problem people. She has been in your office several times before because of an attendance problem. As she sits down, Irene does not return your salutation. She sits there and stares at the floor, ignoring all your questions.

During an interview with someone like Irene, use the following tactics:

1. When it is Irene's turn to speak but she remains silent, lean for-ward and counter with your own silence, accompanied by eye contact and raised eyebrows. Maintain this silent expectant stare for at least 10 seconds. That time interval will seem much longer, and you will feel the urge to renew the conversation sooner. Resist that urge.
2. Finally break silence with, "You have not answered my questions, Irene. Is there some reason for that?" or "What is going on here, Irene? Have I said something to upset you?"
3. If her silence persists, with or without nonverbal responses such as shoulder shrugs or head shakes, do not give up yet. Say, "Irene, I am still waiting." Try the "I guess" approach.[2] For example, "I guess you feel that nobody values what you say" or "I guess you are angry at me because...." Try, "Irene, I need this information from you."
4. If she says, "Can I go now?" reply, "Not yet, Irene, I am still wait-ing for some answers." If she starts to stand up to leave, put out your hand and tell her to sit back down. State the consequences of her remaining silent: "Irene, you may have a good reason for not talking, but this is not beneficial to our relationship. I am very concerned about where this is taking us."
5. If Irene still remains silent, terminate the interview with, "I take it that you are not ready to talk to me, Irene. Since we still must resolve this problem, I want to see you here tomorrow at the same time." Avoid an apologetic or tentative conclusion, and do not thank her for coming in.

During such interviews, you may note a stilted or uncomfortable dialogue during which the other person either hesitates before responding or ignores some of your queries. To get a better conversational flow, start with questions that are of a nonsensitive nature, preferably on a topic of the person's interest. Follow with the more sensitive ones. Another tactic is simply to use multiple open-ended questions. Closed-ended questions are too easy to ignore or can be answered with a slight nod or shake of the head.

The silent bosses pose another set of challenges. Getting the silent treatment from your boss can be intimidating. This silence usually occurs when bosses are reluctant to make decisions or to commit themselves. They may need time to get more information, but they do not want to admit that they do not already have a handle on the problem. They may want to get advice or to avoid the problem by passing the buck. They may be pondering over solutions, formulating the best way to express sensitive issues, or getting their emotions under control.

Obviously, the better you know your boss, the more likely you are to be able to interpret his silence. You can try the expectant stare already described. Do not rush the silent boss. If you sense that the barrier may be lack of understanding, provide more information. If you fail to evoke a response, ask when it would be convenient for you to return. If you now get a verbal response, the return visit will probably be more fruitful. If you do not get a response, pick a time and enunciate it (eg, "I guess I picked a bad time to talk about this, John. If it is okay with you, I will come back first thing tomorrow morning").

Your best action may be to say that you assume that his silence means agreement, and that you will go ahead with your recommendation. Sometimes, at that point, your boss will spring up and shout something like, "You do that and you are fired!" Congratulations, you broke the silence!

THE SUPER-SENSITIVES

Super-sensitive individuals take offense at whatever they perceive to be a put-down. They are extremely sensitive to criticism—often bursting into tears, shouting, or dashing off to the restroom. When this behavior is effective for them, they have a potent tool for manipulating colleagues and superiors.

Solution: Handle super-sensitives with care but do not be manipulated by these reactions. Never withhold negative feedback because of previous over-reactions. Do not apologize for what you said or did. For example:

Supervisor (during counseling session): "Karen, I find it hard to discuss this when you sob like that. Would you like a few minutes to compose yourself?" Supervisor hands Karen a tissue and goes on with his discussion. If Karen, instead of crying, jumps up and runs out of your office, do no run after her or demand that she return. Instead, reschedule the meeting and at that time make no mention of the previous episode. Karen has learned that her inappropriate behavior was not effective. If she loses her temper and starts shouting, wait a minute or so. If she does not calm down, get up and leave your office.

In the case of the weepers, try to establish better rapport. They probably need more moral support than your other employees.

THE MOODY PEOPLE

Most people have some mood swings. It is a matter of degree and circumstances that is important. Transient moodiness, such as that during a grieving period, usually does not require any action by supervisors, but a persistent or markedly depressed state calls for professional help. Between these two extremes are a variety of moods manifested by sorrow, sullenness, irritability, or other personality changes.

Solution: Ignore mild transient moods. If they persist, acknowledge them without agreeing with them. Ask questions and listen with empathy. Do not flood these folks with sympathy. Sympathy may result in the persistence of the moods and possibly lead to the martyr syndrome. Empathy is more effective. If the situation does not improve, suggest professional counseling.

THE NICE PEOPLE WITH MINOR BUT IRRITATING HABITS

Some colleagues have vexatious mannerisms, irritating laughs, bizarre gestures, or other annoying habits. They may have been told about these, but the behavior is so ingrained that they are no longer aware of how irritating it is. Bramson[1] calls this "behavior blindness." These habits are chronic and often persist despite the efforts of spouses and colleagues to effect a change. In some instances the person is aware of what he is doing but continues because it evokes attention. Even though this attention is of the critical variety, for many people it is better to be criticized than to be ignored (eg, the employee who likes to crack his knuckles because it elicits a chorus of groans from the people around him).

Solution: Bramson[1] emphasizes that simply adding to the complaints that others have registered with these offenders seldom gets results. He emphasizes that you must be emphatic about how strongly you feel about the annoying behavior, since casual remarks are not enough. Tell the person that you have something important to talk over with him and set an appointment for later in the day. During the interim, the person will wonder what this important thing is. When you meet and present your feelings, you are more likely to get favorable action than if you make fun of the habit or limit your action to brief comments. Obviously, these have failed in the past.

Whether the habit is done on a conscious or subconscious level, emphasize that you know how difficult it is to break a habit. Suggest that you will help—provided the person accepts this help—by signaling to him in an unobtrusive way when you observe the annoying behavior or hear the offending comment. Occasionally you must take more drastic action such as warning the person that whenever this behavior is manifested you will get up and leave the room or insist that the person do so.

If the problem is one of body odor or bad breath, do not use anonymous notes or surreptitiously leave a bottle of mouthwash on the person's desk. Be direct and honest. If a medical aspect is involved, a physician may have to be consulted.

Suggested verbal responses:

- "Luke, I have a great urge to reprimand you whenever you roll your eyes up when you disagree with me."
- "Sarah, I notice a problem with body odor. I know that I will not have to bring it up again."

THE PEOPLE WITH POOR APPEARANCES

When you confront a person with a poor appearance, ask yourself these key questions: Does the person's appearance offend customers or interfere in the orderly conduct of business (eg, cause people to stop work and stare)? Does it violate any policy or rule? Is it a safety hazard (eg, woolen sweaters in microbiology laboratories can attract bacteria due to static electricity; shoes with high heels are dangerous on slippery or uneven floors). If your answers are "no," or it is simply a matter of differences in taste, you may have to put up with their appearances. However, if "yes" is the answer, you are justified in taking action.

Solution: Try not to hire these people. Those who show up for employment interviews looking like something the cat dragged in are exhibiting their best appearance. If that is not suitable for the job being offered, avoid hiring them.

During orientation of new employees, emphasize the importance of appearance, especially if they have direct contact with customers. Discuss the dress code and your personal expectations. Forewarning is always better than criticizing later. For example:

"Our dress code is fairly lenient, Debbie, but we do have to draw the line at times. Lately, you have been wearing embossed sweaters that have drawn negative comments from some of our physicians and patients. I would appreciate it if your attire was more formal."

THE MESSY ONES

When it comes to messy desks or offices, neatness is in the eyes of the beholder. Before you can get employees to clean up their act, you must convince them that there is a mess. Sometimes, fastidious supervisors make a big fuss over a little disorder. The key point is whether a disorderly desk or work area has a negative effect on performance, coworkers, or customers. A receptionist's desk in full view of visitors is not the same as a desk in the corner of the maintenance department.

Solution: To get people to clean up their space, you must prove that it is necessary. Sometimes it is best to compromise. For example:

> Supervisor: "Alan, please keep your desk free of all those stacks of papers, books, and journals."
> Alan: "Why? I can find everything on my desk."
> Supervisor: "Alan, I know you can, but others have to find reports that are on your desk when you are not around, and they complain that they waste a lot of time looking for the reports."
> Alan: "Would you get off my case if I put an outgoing box for reports on my credenza?"
> Supervisor: "Okay, Alan, that would be fine, and thanks for your cooperation."

Some barriers may be beyond the employee's control (eg, when visiting VIPs drop their coats on a receptionist's chair or delivery people place large cartons in doorways). Help your staffers to eliminate such barriers.

THE PEOPLE WHO USE OFFENSIVE LANGUAGE

Sexual language must never to be tolerated (see chapter 25 on sexual harassment). Sexist and racist remarks or profanity should not go unchallenged. For example:

> (Sexist remark)
> Female physician (after a patient in the emergency room demands that he be seen by a "real doctor—a man"): "Sir, that demand is sexist, and I do not like it. You probably did not realize that I am a physician. Now, what can I do for you?"
> (Profanity)
> Supervisor after Bart has just let loose a series of four-letter words: "Bart, that is the last time I want to hear that kind of language here."
> Bart: "I thought this was a free country. What about my freedom of speech?"

Supervisor: "That is not freedom of speech, that is gutter talk, and it has no place in a professional organization. Knock it off."

THE JEALOUS COWORKERS

Envy, which is wishing you had what someone else has, is natural. Jealousy is envy loaded with feelings of ill will toward others. Such feelings are common when employees compete for promotion or recognition. Frustrated people may try to undermine your position by starting ill-founded rumors, publicly berating you, causing a bottleneck, or turning others against you. When any of these disloyal activities occur, you must take firm action.

Solution: Discuss the problem with your boss and get his support. Then, confront the jealous one. Lay it on the line. Say what you have seen or heard and that you want it stopped. Describe your future expectations (eg, "I do not want arguments in front of staff, patients, or physicians. If you have a gripe, see me in my office").

If the undesired behavior persists, remind the person that it will affect his next performance rating, assignments, special privileges, such as approval for attending meetings, and possibly continued employment.

If the person berates you in public, it is sometimes best to ignore the remarks. At other times you must respond. If an employee criticizes you in front of your boss, turn to your boss and say, "Of course I have a response to that, but I prefer not make a public spectacle of it. I will brief you later in your office." Now, your accuser is stopped cold and has no idea what you are going to say to the boss.

THE INCESSANT TALKERS AND SOCIALIZERS

Talkers and socializers suffer from verbal diarrhea. Monday morning finds them rehashing weekend sports or their recreational activities. They repeat their broadcasts as long as they find listeners. You must know how to act when these time-wasters cause bottlenecks.

Solution: Break up the little group discussions in the hallway. Give the verbose ones extra assignments. When they learn that too much talk and too little work results in extra assignments, they will modify their abuse of time. If possible, isolate them from willing ears. Encourage them to do their socializing during breaks. (See chapter 14 for advice on how to cut them off at meetings.)

THE EMPLOYEES WHO TRY TO DUMP ON YOU

Upward dumping ("reverse delegation") is a form of manipulation in which subordinates try to get supervisors or colleagues to do their work. Nurse

Jack hates to tinker with the traction apparatus on orthopedic beds. Whenever one of these set-ups gets messed up, he calls for the supervisor. When Specialist Lynn appears, Nurse Jack mumbles something about other duties and rushes off. Lynn should call him back and insist that he watch how to hook up all the ropes and pulleys so he can do it himself the next time.

THE EMPLOYEES WHO GO OVER YOUR HEAD

Ideally, your boss will send these complainers and snitchers right back to you after he realizes that the employee has not given you an opportunity to respond. Unfortunately, some managers are all too willing to lend an ear to employees who bypass their supervisors—especially when the manager and the supervisor do not get along.

Solution: As soon as you become aware of this situation, confront your boss. Relate exactly what you have observed or have been told. Correct inaccuracies and pinpoint outright lies. Plead with your boss to give you an opportunity to respond each time to what these employees articulate. Encourage the boss to send for you on these occasions so that you can respond in front of the person. Describe how these undercover operations affect your department and your state of mind. Let the employee know that you know what is going on and how you feel about it. Illustrate how such activities are counterproductive and will ultimately backfire.

THE TWO EMPLOYEES WHO ARE FEUDING

Two people may not get along at work for many reasons. In addition to differences in race, nationality, religion, age, politics, and gender, they may be competing for attention, promotion, recognition, turf, or limited resources. Personality differences get blamed most often. Sometimes bystanders provoke the situation.

Before you attribute the problem to personality clashes, look for external causes. For instance, ambiguous position descriptions may not indicate who does what responsibility or who has what authority.

Solution: Supervisors have three options from which to choose:

Avoidance. This is best when it is not your problem or you lack the authority to act.

Arbitrate. This is analyzing the situation and then taking sides or dictating a solution. This approach often fails, and serious side effects can result. For example: The nurse and physician's assistant constantly argue over who should answer medical questions from patients. You decide that the physician's assistant should. You rewrite their position descriptions and explain to each how you arrived at that decision.

Mediate. You encourage the pair to solve their own problem, keep the pair from exploding, and guide them into mutually agreeable solutions. Here you must be perceived as neutral by both parties. You may not take sides. Sometimes the problem is solved simply by telling the duo that they do not have to like each other to work together, but that you expect them to act as adults and to treat each other civilly on the job. If that approach does not work, your goal is to talk to each person individually, looking for an underlying cause of the problem. A solution may emerge during one of these conversations. Job redesign, clarification of limits of authority, or revising territorial boundaries may provide the remedy. If the problem is still not solved, hold a joint meeting. The intent of this meeting is to convert them from adversaries to problem-solvers. Follow this sequence:

1. Warn them that if they do not work out a solution, administrative action will be taken—action that will not please either party.
2. Seek some common ground or area of agreement (eg, "You both agree that our goal is to improve customer service, right?").
3. Lay out the ground rules for the meeting, like a debate: "First, Kevin will have his say without any interruptions. Make no personal attacks. Then Bill will ask any questions about what Kevin said and will summarize Kevin's argument. Then the process will be reversed."
4. Listen to both sides impartially. Make them abide by the rules. Do not tolerate interruptions, blaming, or name calling. Make each person summarize what the other person said to clarify any miscommunications. Ask each person what he wants changed.
5. If they clam up, become a spokesperson: "Stop me if I am wrong, but I think that what Kathy wants is.... Is that right, Kathy?"
6. Review areas of agreement and disagreement.
7. Discuss the pros and cons of each alternative and get them to agree to one.
8. Clarify future behavior: "What are we going to do differently?" "What are we going to do if...?"
9. Congratulate them for reaching an agreement. Say that you have confidence in them resolving their differences.
10. Follow up. Hold additional sessions if necessary.

If they cannot solve their differences, you must decide if you can live with the flawed situation. If not, take whatever administrative action is necessary (eg, to reassign them so they no longer work together).

Suggested verbal responses to feuding employees:

- "This behavior is unacceptable. Each of you is too valuable for me to allow it to continue."
- "You agree that each of you is competent and interested in providing excellent patient care, right? Good!"

- "Stop the name calling. Stick to the facts."
- "Now, tell me exactly what you want the other person to do."
- "Margaret, is that really what you think Will is saying?" "Is that what you have been saying, Will?" "Margaret, as I understand it, you would like Will to…, right?" "Will, you would like Margaret to stop…, right?"
- "Congratulations. I think you have solved this problem. Now, let's go out and make it work."

THE GOSSIPS

The GOSSIP thrives on creating and spreading rumors about other employees. While a little benign gossip is harmless, something must be done when character is attacked or misinformation affects work or morale.

The GOSSIP wants attention, so supply it in healthy ways. Spike misinformation by insisting on validation or correcting false comments. Explain how gossiping is having an adverse effect on the work team and that people are withholding information from him because they fear that what they say will be repeated in distorted forms. Do not encourage the GOSSIP by reacting positively to his messages. In some instances, it is necessary to shun these people.

THE CONCEALERS

The CONCEALER likes the powerful feeling of withholding information that other employees need. Their colleagues react by doing the same. The result is that work and morale are affected. Try to find the motivation behind the lack of communication. Confront the person when you know that important information is being withheld, and praise him when he is more open. Sometimes CONCEALERS respond favorably when they are given training or leadership roles, but be careful when you try the latter. Unless these individuals show evidence of becoming more open in their communication, they will perform poorly in any leadership role. Increased authority plus their unwillingness to share information can pose a threatening situation for the supervisor and other members of the work team.

REFERENCES

1. Bramson RM. *Coping With Difficult People*. New York, NY: Random House; 1981.

2. Brinkman R, Kirschner R. *How to Deal With Difficult People* [videotapes]. Boulder, Colo: CareerTrack Publications; 1991.

24. Hostile People

Hostile people have one thing in common: they attack you and your self-esteem. What distinguishes them is how they go about achieving this goal. These people play hard ball. Their theme is, "I win, you lose."

The psychopathology of hostility is beyond the scope of this discussion. Suffice it to say that some HOSTILES see interpersonal relationships as game playing in which their opponents are always the losers. In fact, many of their dialogues can be found among the examples of psychological games described in treatises on transactional analysis.[1]

The "big three" hostiles are called SHERMAN TANKS, EXPLODERS, and SNIPERS by Bramson,[2] whose terminology will be used in this chapter. Readers are strongly urged to read Bramson's original work—it is a classic.

In this chapter, I will provide assertive responses to hostile attacks, which in some instances you may wish to use verbatim. However, the exact words you use will depend on your individual interactive style and vocabulary. Whatever the phrases are, they are more effective if they are formulated and rehearsed before your next encounter with a HOSTILE. Even better, role-play them with a spouse or trusted colleague.

Your unspoken assertive message to HOSTILES is that you respect their right to have feelings and to speak their minds, but that you also have those same rights. In addition, regardless of the rank and power of the hostile person, you do not have to listen to profane, intimidating, offensive, or obnoxious language.

Two requisites are needed to achieve this goal of freedom of expression: a modicum of self-esteem and some robust assertiveness. That is why these two vital communication tools were discussed early on in this book. If you are nonassertive, none of the advice provided here will be of any value; your passivity will prevent you from using it. Your recourse is to enroll in a class on assertiveness, seek counseling advice, or refer to other audiotapes or publications (see references and suggested readings at the conclusion of chapter 3).

Before we look in on some of these hostile people, remember that the power of communication comes not so much from words as from nonverbal language. Over one half of the power of communication comes from kinetics (body language) and over one third from voice tone and volume. The words themselves provide less than one tenth of the power.[3] Therefore, what the other person sees and the strength of your voice are critical factors. For example, if you are under attack from a hostile person and you speak in a soft, timid voice while looking down at the ground, you have lost.

SHERMAN TANKS

Of all the hostiles, SHERMAN TANKS are the most difficult to handle because they often have power, they usually are professionally or administratively competent, and they know exactly what it is that they want. SHERMAN TANKS (Bullies, Dictators, Steam Rollers) have had years of successful intimidation. Their victims are too numerous to count.

SHERMAN TANKS may be superiors, customers, inspectors, staff coordinators, or even colleagues. Every executive suite and medical staff has at least one.

SHERMAN TANKS are results-oriented with a dash of sadism. In other words, they know what they want from their victims, but in addition, they enjoy the discomfort they inflict while getting their own wants or needs addressed. They have permanently adopted this style because it is so effective. They may be physically intimidating and are always psychologically threatening. They are aggressive, abrupt, arrogant, and autocratic. They are contemptuous of their victims. When they attack, they expect their targets either to fight back (aggression) or to capitulate (passivity).

Evidence of rage or weakness by their victims stimulates SHERMAN TANKS to push on. A victim may win a battle but usually will lose the war. Defeat does not cure these difficult people—it leaves them seething and plotting, sometimes converting them into SNIPERS.[2]

The most successful strategy is assertiveness—to stand up to them but without fighting. When possible, avoid confrontations when your self-confidence is low. Unfortunately, these individuals often seem to materialize from nowhere, taking you by surprise. One of the advantages of a local personal network is that you are often alerted that one of these SHERMAN TANKS is heading toward your department.

In any confrontation you must be assertive enough to get their attention and then state your own opinions and perceptions while remaining emotionally neutral. When they launch into a tirade, do not get defensive or try to counterattack.

How to Cope With Sherman Tanks

1. *Hear them out.*
   - Hold your ground. Equalize eye level as much as possible. Ask them to sit down. Stand up if they refuse to be seated.
   - Maintain eye contact, but do not try to stare them down.
   - Hold yourself erect. Do not hunch your shoulders, back up, or cower.
   - Allow them to vent feelings without interruption.
   - Take some deep breaths. This provides better cerebral oxygenation, helps you to feel in control, and modulates your emotional reaction.[4]
   - When they pause for breath say, "I disagree, but go on."
   - Instead of counterattacking, urge them to continue or ask some open-ended questions. Get it all out.
   - Concentrate on what they are saying. Backtrack by paraphrasing (eg, "What you are saying is.... Is that right?" or "You think that...?"

2. *Respond nondefensively.*
   - When they start repeating, break in with a "Pardon me," then reply. If they continue, wave your hands to get their attention and call out their name loudly.
   - Turn up your voice volume sufficiently to be heard, but not as loud as theirs. Your voice must be neither plaintive nor belligerent.
   - Insist that they listen to your response. Each time they interrupt, say, "You interrupted me," and go on. Do not incur their wrath by trying to deliver a lecture on interruptions.
   - Be tentative or noncommittal. Use phrases such as, "it appears," "it seems," "perhaps," or "possibly."

3. *Switch to solving the problem that brought them in.*
   - Remember that their behavior was intended not only to humble you, but also to get something done. Now that you have taken the fun out of the former, they are ready to discuss the problem. If they are right, apologize briefly and move to a solution as quickly as possible (eg, "You are right, and here is what I'm going to do"); or ask them what they think should be done.

Suggested verbal responses:

- "I understand your point of view, but I disagree."
- "I agree with much of what you said, but I must point out that…"
- "You have said a number of things, and I do not agree with some of them. If I heard you right, you think…, correct?"
- "I did not interrupt you and would appreciate it if you allowed me to respond."
- "Excuse me, but you are interrupting."
- "Possibly you were misinformed about what we did."
- "It appears that we could have…."
- "Perhaps we can find a solution that satisfies both of us."
- "Maybe we can get around that regulation by…."
- "We do not condone that kind of abuse here."

Six Important Don'ts

1. Don't panic. Keep cool.
2. Don't interrupt.
3. Don't accuse them of anything.
4. Don't complain or whine.
5. Don't argue. Stick to the facts.
6. Don't put up with offensive language or profanity. Walk away. If the person has much influence or power, tell your boss what you did and why.

How to Handle a Sherman Tank Who is a Customer

Expect occasional SHERMAN TANKS and be ready for them. These folks are repeaters. Learn from previous attacks or from warnings you get from your colleagues.[5]

- Listen, listen, listen—patiently, without interrupting.
- Do not blame policy or administration. Customers are often infuriated at such buck passing.
- Briefly explain what happened but do not go into great detail or recite a litany of excuses. Customers do not want to hear about computer breakdowns or backorders—they want action.
- Ask them what they want done. Grant that request if you can and state when it will be accomplished. If you cannot oblige, say what you will do.

- If they want to see your boss, say that they have that right, but you would like to solve the problem for them without any further delay. Do not look perturbed over the person's demand.

EXPLODERS

EXPLODERS (Volcanos, Erupters, Grenades, Time Bombs), like SHER-MAN TANKS, manifest anger but with significant differences. SHERMAN TANKS always exhibit the same overbearing attitude, whereas EXPLODERS are gentle between attacks. The anger of SHERMAN TANKS is contrived and under their complete control; the anger of EXPLODERS is real and partially-to-completely out of control. EXPLODERS sometimes push or strike others.

The EXPLODER is an adult who suffers from childlike temper tantrums. In fact, Bramson's studies have shown that many EXPLODERS, when they were young children, discovered that losing their tempers was often the only way to get what they wanted. EXPLODERS, too, found that people often do not take them seriously unless they "get mad."

These time bombs have a tremendous need for respect. They explode when their self-esteem is threatened, when they are the target of a joke, when they are kept waiting, when they are ignored, or when their competency is questioned.

Your goal is to bring them back to their senses as quickly as possible.[4] Coping is a matter of helping them regain self-control. Give them time to run down. EXPLODERS are like wind-up toys—they wind down if you can wait them out. After their explosion, they may become pussy cats. They are often very apologetic and may break down and weep.

Some of these people get through the worst of their explosions very quickly. Your task is to douse the fire and get their attention. If an EXPLODER appears to be out of control, respond as you would to a hysterical person. In a loud voice call out, "Stop! Stop!" or "Okay! Okay!" or keep repeating her name. Wave your arms to get her attention.

A clever tactic is to say that you need a notebook to write down what the EXPLODER is saying because it is very important. This buys still more time for her to wind down, and it also boosts her self-esteem.

If she continues to rant and rave, her voice will be loud and fast. Say that you cannot write quickly enough when she speaks so fast; she must slow down. As soon as she slows down, the pitch and volume of her voice also plummets. Anger drains away. Often she will now sit down for the first time.

Listen carefully for two essentials: (1) what is setting them off, their "hot button," and (2) what it is that they want. You may hear a word clue that is repeated over and over, such as "policy," "schedules," "recognition," or "consideration." A part-time laboratory technician might say, "Laboratory administration thinks that we are stupid," to which a laboratory manager responds, "We do not think that part-timers are stupid, absolutely not."

Do not try to explain things while an EXPLODER is still upset—her listening mechanism is out of order. After she has calmed down and becomes rational, find out exactly what she wants. Use her name frequently. If an apology is in order, make it, but add that you did not like the way she conducted herself. Show that you are intent on helping by stating what you intend to do.

If you do not know what started the outburst, try repeating, "There must be a misunderstanding, and it does not have to be this way."[4]

If she remains irrational, say loudly that you want to help but not when she is in such a state. Call a break (eg, "Julie, let's take a 15-minute break. I will come back after we have both calmed down") or leave immediately if she becomes verbally or physically abusive. Say that you will talk to her later.

If people explode over the telephone and you cannot break into the conversation, try remaining completely silent. When the volatile person "hears" only silence coming back over the line, she will usually lower her voice and ask if anyone is there—thinking that you may have hung up. The lowering of her voice will dissipate some of the anger. You quietly respond: "Yes, I am still listening." Then use that opportunity to wedge in your response. If you discover what her trigger mechanism is, try to avoid it in the future.

Suggested verbal responses:

- "Could you run that by me a little slower?"
- "I want to hear everything you have to say, but not like this. I will get back to you later."
- "I apologize for…, but I do not like being called names or being yelled at."
- "I am sorry to be rude, Bob, (interrupting) but we seem to be repeating ourselves. I am out of alternatives. The best I can do is…."[5]

Six Important Don'ts

1. Don't try to reason with them when they are irrational.
2. Don't walk out on them unless they are abusive. Leaving the scene deprives them of the respect they need so much.
3. Don't yell back insults or defensive remarks. Do shout their name or repetitive statements to get their attention.
4. Don't get involved in a verbal boxing match in which accusations or threats swing wildly back and forth without any attempt at compromise.
5. Don't try to persuade an angry person to change the subject. When a person is that emotionally upset, her mind cannot be turned to another topic.

6. Don't forgive them for their behavior, even when they return all apologetic. Forgiveness reinforces the explosive behavior.
Repeat, "I am always willing to listen to you, but not like that."

How to Handle an Exploder Who is a Subordinate

Some employees have an explosive temper on a short fuse, and they become angry at the slightest provocation. These individuals often are job-hoppers. They stay on a job only until they blow up, tell the boss off, and quit or get fired. Emotional immaturity, low self-esteem, and marginal competence are characteristic of these firecrackers. They have intense feelings of frustration, fear, prejudice, or guilt.

Thorough employment screening usually weeds out these people. If you are stuck with one, keep her away from customers. EXPLODERS can do a lot of damage. Do not take personally what they say in fits of temper. Reply with, "I am sorry you said that. I would think that over if I were you. You have nothing to gain by offending me." If the session continues to degenerate, end it. Do not judge, criticize, or moralize, just end it. Simply say that the interview is no longer productive, and you will meet again later. Get up and move toward your door.

In my experience, professional counseling is not often helpful in chronic cases, but it is worth recommending. More often these employees are terminated via the disciplinary route. If they resign during one of their rages, do not let them change their minds.

SNIPERS

SNIPERS (Foxes, Saboteurs, Needlers) would like to be in control, like SHERMAN TANKS, but they lack the courage. The SNIPERS' weapons are sarcasm, snide remarks, and sick humor.[4] "They throw snowballs with rocks in them."[2] SNIPERS have discovered that masquerading sharp, stinging remarks lets them get away with attacking you without assuming any responsibility. They do most of their dirty work in front of other people who provide their cover.[6]

SNIPERS utilize innuendoes, sotto voce remarks, not-too-subtle digs, and nonplayful kidding. Their remarks usually drip with sarcasm. Their assaults are not always carried out in your presence. They often talk behind your back, knowing that what they say will reach you. When you respond angrily, they retort, "Can't you take a joke?" "I was only kidding," or "Where is your sense of humor?"

SNIPERS' victims tend not to fight back because they do not want to make a scene. They smile weakly, wonder what is going on, and later find out that they have taken some hits. They lie awake nights thinking of what they should have said or done.[2]

How to Cope With Snipers

Your goal is to flush them out and defang them.[4] Recognize the zingers when you hear them. Say to yourself, "Well, here comes one of Andrea's little zingers." Do not laugh, even if it is a little funny or all the other people giggle or snicker. But do not ignore it either.

Bypass your sense of politeness. Immediately stop what you are doing or saying, turn toward the SNIPER, and repeat exactly what you heard—these "jokes" lose their punch when repeated.[4] Then say, "Andrea, that seemed to be a barb aimed at me. Is that what it was?" or "Are you making fun of what I just said?"[2]

As soon as you have called her on this, you have blown her cover. Now she must either confirm what she said or try to weasel out of it with something like, "Where is your sense of humor?" Respond with a sour smile, "Well, it did not sound funny to me."[4]

If she backs up what she said, you may learn something important. Critical feedback can be worthwhile. If she backs down, you have turned the tables on her.

Alternatively, ask the SNIPER what her remark has to do with the subject under discussion (the "relevance question") or what was the purpose of the remark (the "intent question").

Ask for help from your associates. When you overhear the SNIPER say, "What a stupid idea. She is still in a dream world," say to the group, "Does anyone else see it that way?" If the SNIPERS' criticism gets support, you can search for more information about it. If the others do not agree, follow with, "I guess we have a difference of opinion" (not "See, you are wrong").[2]

If the SNIPER suddenly becomes a SHERMAN TANK, go into your TANK defense.[4]

After a "snowball throwing" meeting, get the SNIPER aside and make a direct accusation. SNIPERS do not function well in one-on-one situations—their camouflage is missing. Do not buy their, "Oh, you are just too sensitive" remarks. Reply that you enjoy a good joke like everyone else, but that what you are hearing are not good jokes.

Suggested verbal responses:

- "Are you trying to make me feel bad?"
- "I know that you do not mean to hurt my feelings, but those remarks do just that. Please stop."
- "I am hearing some third-hand remarks attributed to you. The latest is…. Did you say that?"
- "I am getting tired of listening to all these little digs during our meetings. If you do not stop, I am going to ask you to stop coming to these sessions."

- "When you have something to say to or about me, please say it directly to me instead of behind my back."
- "What did you mean when you turned your thumbs down (rolled up your eyes, smirked, etc) while I was making my presentation?"

How to Handle a Sniper Who is Passive Aggressive

PASSIVE AGGRESSIVES represent a subset of the SNIPER. Like SNIPERS, they conceal their antagonism. This term does not mean that these people are passive one moment and aggressive the next. Wetzler[7] aptly calls this behavior "sugar-coated hostility." PASSIVE AGGRESSIVES are manipulators who pretend to be helpless while they infuriate their superiors and associates. They represent attempts by the weak to thwart authority.[7]

PASSIVE AGGRESSIVES lack the confidence to challenge authority directly, so their resistance comes out indirectly and covertly. They believe that they are getting a raw deal—often regarding their bosses as dictators who have reduced them to hapless, powerless victims of excessive demands by others, thus causing them to feel angry and resentful.

PASSIVE AGGRESSIVES play many of the psychological games described by Berne.[1] These include the games of "Kick Me," "Schlemiel," and "Wooden leg" (see chapter 11). Typical things they do to try your patience are to show up late for a meeting or to submit late reports, to get angry with you but refuse to tell you why, or to foul up a procedure. They apologize superficially, give you endless excuses, or just clam up. Inwardly they enjoy your anger or discomfort.

You are not likely to change their personalities, which may even be resistant to psychiatric help. Your goal is to insist on behavior that meets your expectations and not to let them upset you when they play their mean psychological games. Do not accept their excuses and never exhibit the anger or frustration you feel.

REFERENCES

1. Berne E. *Games People Play: The Psychology of Human Relationships*. New York, NY: Grove Press; 1964.

2. Bramson RM. *Coping With Difficult People*. New York, NY: Random House; 1981.

3. Mehrabian R. *Nonverbal Communication*. New York, NY: Addline-Atherton Publishers; 1972.

4. Brinkman R, Kirschner R. *How to Deal With Difficult People* [videotape]. Boulder, Colo: CareerTrack Publications; 1988.

5. Tucker RK. *Fighting it Out With Difficult People*. Dubuque, Iowa: Kendall/Hunt Publishers; 1987.

6. Solomon M. *Working With Difficult People*. Englewood Cliffs, NJ: Prentice Hall; 1990.

7. Wetzler S. Sugar-coated hostility. *Newsweek*. October 12, 1992:14.

25.   Sexual Harassment

Sexual harassment is defined as "unwelcome behavior of a sexual nature or with sexual overtones." In 1980, the Equal Employment Opportunity Commission (EEOC) developed guidelines defining sexual harassment as a form of gender discrimination and, therefore, a violation of Title VII of the Civil Rights Act of 1964.[1]

THE THREE FORMS OF SEXUAL HARASSMENT

Quid Pro Quo

Quid pro quo (something for something) occurs when an employee is expected to grant unwanted sexual demands or suffer the loss of some tangible job benefit such as promotion, salary increase, preferred assignment, special perks, or keeping the job. It does not matter if this coercion takes place at work or outside the workplace. Frequently, a single incident of quid pro quo harassment merits disciplinary action.[2]

Hostile Work Environment

In a hostile work environment, unwelcome sexual conduct interferes with a person's job performance or is intimidating or offensive. This behavior is considered harassment even if it leads to no tangible or economic consequences. Sexually hostile activities can be verbal, visual, or tactile. *Verbal* abuse includes sexual language, innuendoes, epithets, or jokes. Sexual letters or phone calls are mentioned frequently. *Visual* offenses consist of provocative gestures, sexually oriented posters, and graffiti on restroom walls. *Tactile* harassment can be sexually oriented touching, patting, pinching, rubbing, or pressing. Because harassment is highly subjective, mistaken intentions can result in inappropriate charges. Friendliness, thoughtlessness, or innocent remarks and bids for attention can be misread.[2] According to the EEOC, a single incident or isolated incidents of offensive sexual conduct or remarks seldom create an abusive environment.

Sexual Favoritism or "Paramour Preference"

Workers can allege sexual harassment by showing that they were denied a chance at promotion because a coworker who had submitted to unwelcome sexual requests from a supervisor was granted the promotion. Similar charges may be brought when management personnel regularly solicit sexual favors from subordinate employees (EEOC Policy Guidance N-915.048, January 1990).

SEXUAL HARASSMENT IS RAMPANT

A study by the U.S. Merit System Protection Board of federal employees found that 42% of all women and 14% of all men who responded had experienced some form of unwanted and uninvited sexual attention.[3] Ringel[4] conducted a national survey of female laboratorians regarding the issue of sexual harassment. Of the respondents, 30% claimed that they had been sexually harassed. Of that group, only one third of the victims reported the harassment; 21% quit their jobs; and in 20% of the reported cases the harassment continued.

WHO ARE THE HARASSERS?

While the majority of charges are made by women against men, women may accuse other women, and men may bring charges against members of either sex. In Ringel's survey of clinical laboratories, 81% of the harassing was done by individuals who had some power over their victims.[4] Coworkers comprise the second largest group of harassers.

SEXUAL HARASSMENT POLICIES AND ENFORCEMENT

Employers are responsible for protecting employees, visitors, and anyone else on the premises from sexual harassment. Failure to do so can result in huge litigation costs. In addition, the employer may experience a decrease in productivity and morale, an increase in absenteeism and turnover, and a negative public perception.[5]

Organizations must promulgate specific policies for sexual harassment. A statement such as, "Sexual harassment will not be tolerated," is totally inadequate. According to one source,[6] a policy should:

- State that sexual harassment will not be tolerated.
- Define quid pro quo and hostile environment harassment.
- Identify employee and management responsibilities.
- Outline a procedure for employees to make complaints about sexual harassment to a person with authority to resolve the complaint.
- Guarantee that all complaints will be treated confidentially.
- Guarantee that employees who complain will not suffer adverse job consequences as a result of the complaint.
- State that any employee who engages in sexual harassment is subject to discipline up to and including discharge.

The policy must be explicit. It must define and give examples of behavior that constitutes sexual harassment and will not be tolerated. For example, employees are prohibited from displaying sexually provocative posters in work areas. Employees who tell sexually explicit jokes or who use sexual profanity or epithets violate standards of behavior.

The Information Must be Communicated Widely

It is not enough to simply formulate a policy. That policy must be made crystal clear to every employee. Most employees know that making job benefits contingent on the granting of sexual favors is sexual harassment (quid pro quo), but they may not realize that sexual jokes, posters, or gestures are also forms of harassment (hostile environment).

Communication can take many forms. Copies of the policy should be included in employee handbooks, posted on bulletin boards, and reprinted periodically in employee newsletters. Group discussions centered around vignettes depicting a wide range of behaviors provide an excellent modality for heightening awareness of prohibited behavior.[3] Guest speakers are readily available and local units of the EEOC or local human relations commissions usually provide free brochures. Videotapes on the subject are ideal educational modalities.

Grievance Procedures

Employers must develop a grievance procedure for sexual harassment that encourages employees to report problems. The traditional procedure for filing other kinds of complaints is unsatisfactory because it calls for a grievance being submitted first to the employee's immediate supervisor, who may be the harasser. The procedure for receiving and investigating complaints must be prompt, fair, and confidential. A complainant must be able to talk to an individual whom he or she trusts.

Development of a policy prohibiting sexual harassment and the availability of a grievance procedure for reporting complaints are not sufficient protection from liability. The courts look instead to the specificity of the policy, the likelihood that grievance procedures will be used, and the adequacy of the organization's response to complaints.[3]

Investigation of Complaints

The single biggest mistake managers make is failing to take every complaint seriously. All complaints must be investigated.[6] Managers must maintain the same sensitivity toward sexual harassment as they do toward discrimination against minorities of race, color, and religion.

It is essential that every supervisor be aware of the policies and procedures relating to sexual harassment and enforce them vigorously and with sensitivity, while not forgetting the rights of the alleged harasser. Obviously, supervisors must avoid any behavior on their part that could be construed as sexual harassment.

The victim is entitled to a fair hearing, but so is the alleged harasser. Complaint investigation involves delicate interpersonal problem solving. Only those individuals with a genuine need to know should have access to the grievance.

Charges of sexual harassment are more likely to be sustained when the complainant: (1) had never given the alleged harasser reason to believe that sexual advances were welcome; (2) had communicated displeasure to the alleged harasser in a forceful way; and (3) registered a formal complaint at the time the harassment occurred, or not too long after it stopped.

Note: Some cases are accepted by EEOC even several years after the alleged violations and after the harassed person had resigned.[2]

STEP-BY-STEP PROCEDURE FOR ADDRESSING COMPLAINTS

1. Listen carefully to the complaint. Insist on specificity. Ask the accuser to document dates, places, names of witnesses, and the

exact statements or behavior of the alleged harasser. Record how long this behavior has been going on and how frequently it occurs. Find out what the alleged victim expects or wants you to do. Do not ask leading questions such as "Do you want a transfer?"

Note: Legal advisors warn that if a complainant later wants to withdraw the charge—usually because of fear of retaliation— you should tell that person that the investigation must continue because a law may have been broken and it is your legal responsibility to continue the investigation. If your organization permits employees to withdraw charges, make sure that you get that decision in writing and duly witnessed.

2. Investigate as soon as possible in accordance with the protocol outlined in the policy of your organization. This usually includes interviewing witnesses and other alleged victims.

3. Confront the harasser with the complaint. Be objective and unbiased. Keep each allegation separate and ask for a response to each one separately. Listen carefully to the rebuttal. Often you find that the accused persons simply are not aware that what they are doing constitutes sexual harassment. If appropriate, state emphatically that this behavior must stop immediately. State the possible consequences if the behavior continues.

4. Document all meetings.

5. After you have met with all parties, get back to the complainant and relate what happened. If no supporting evidence is found, explain this. Reaffirm the commitment on your part and that of the organization to prevent sexual harassment. Review what is necessary to sustain charges. If you substantiated the charge and took action, inform the complainant of this and ask him to report any additional violations immediately.

6. Monitor the situation. If harassment continues, discuss possible additional remedial measures with your immediate supervisor.

Remedial Actions

Management must take the following three remedial steps when a grievance of sexual harassment is filed.[6]

1. Stop the harassment.

2. Address the victim's needs by restoring any job benefits or opportunities that were lost because of the harassment. In some cases, professional counseling may be needed to overcome the stress caused by the harassment.

3. Discipline the harasser.

Sanctions Against Harassers

Sanctions include verbal or written warnings or reprimands, probation, demotion, suspension, letters placed in personnel files, demotions, suspension, or dismissals. The action varies according to each institution's protocol. Uniformity of action is imperative.

When the appropriate action is to separate the parties, the transfer should not appear to disadvantage the harassed person. If a less desirable position is awarded, management may be perceived as retaliating against the victim for making the complaint.[6]

WHEN YOU ARE THE TARGET OF A SEXUAL HARASSER

1. Do not encourage the person to act or behave in ways that you find objectionable. Reject any unwelcome advances or propositions. Change the subject when a conversation turns to sexual topics. Do not laugh or smile when off-color stories are told. Walk away or object to what you hear or see.
2. Explain that you want only a professional relationship. Refer to the examples of responses given below. Repeat such responses each time an incident occurs, expressing your disapproval more strongly each time. Meanwhile, review the personnel policy regarding sexual harassment or seek the advice of a senior member of the human resources department.
3. Warn the offender that if he or she persists, you will regard the activities as sexual harassment and will report them. It is a matter of individual judgment to determine how much you should tolerate before blowing the whistle. Remember that it is often the victim who suffers the most after registering a complaint. Without the support of witnesses or, in the case of hostile environment charges, lack of agreement that working conditions are abusive, the victim may be perceived by coworkers as being prudish or trying to make trouble for the boss. Unfortunately, in some instances upper management is not supportive and may even be hostile toward those who make charges of sexual harassment.
4. Document each episode. Get witnesses if possible. Remember that a single incident rarely suffices to make a case.
5. If you filed a complaint and feel that it was not handled to your satisfaction, notify the human resources department that you intend to file a grievance with the local EEOC representative or contact a legal service agency, state discrimination agency, or a lawyer. If you have a union, complain to your union representative. When legal action is threatened, bureaucrats run scared.
6. If you are still dissatisfied, do what you threatened to do.

Appropriate Verbal Responses to a Potential Harasser

We should not tolerate any more harassment from people who have authority or influence over us than we do from those who have less power over us. However, the recommended language used should be appropriate to the individual. Following are some examples:

- "I prefer to keep our relationship on a strictly professional basis."
- "When you put your arm around my waist, Doctor, it makes me very uncomfortable. Please do not do it anymore."
- "Keep your hands to yourself."
- "Stop telling those off-color stories."
- "One more comment about any part of my anatomy, and I will charge you with sexual harassment."

REFERENCES

1. Discrimination because of sex under Title VII of the Civil Rights Act of 1964 as amended: adoption of final interpretive guidelines. U.S. Equal Employment Opportunity Commission Part 1604. *Federal Register.* November 10, 1980.
2. Weiss DH. *Fair, Square and Legal.* New York, NY: AMACOM; 1991.
3. Lewis KE, Johnson PR. Preventing sexual harassment complaints based on hostile work environments. *SAM Adv Manage J.* Spring 1991:21-26.
4. Ringel MJ. Parenthood, harassment, and other workplace distractions. *MLO.* 1992;24:29-33.
5. Kandel WL. Current development in employment litigation. *Employ Rel Law J.* 1988;14:439-451.
6. *Sexual Harassment Manual For Managers and Supervisors.* Chicago, Ill: Commerce Clearing House, Inc; 1991.

26.   Romances in the Workplace

I t is only natural that people who work together may become romantically involved. Most of us would agree that shared work interests, the opportunity to observe each other under fire, and mutual interactions with many different people provide stronger foundations for significant relationships than do casual meetings elsewhere (eg, in singles' bars). In fact, the work arena is one of the very best places to meet a future spouse. Nevertheless, romances at work can wreak havoc for the lovers and their bosses. This is particularly true if: (1) one of the duo is married to someone else; (2) it is a boss-subordinate relationship; (3) it is a romantic triangle on the job; or (4) the organization has a policy that prohibits such activities.

When a romance becomes a cause of concern, people expect the boss to do something about it.[1] This is something of a paradox because another traditional belief holds that managers should not get involved in the private lives of their subordinates.[2]

PROBLEMS CAUSED BY ROMANCES AT WORK

Poor Time Management by Romantic Couple

Such problems might include long lunches and breaks, work hours adjusted to suit the couple rather than the department, and mental and physical preoccupation with the other person.

Interest Shifts From Teamwork to Each Other

The affair may undermine the power relationships within the worker group. Tension may develop between the romantic couple and their fellow workers, especially if their inappropriate public displays of affection or extramarital liaisons are frowned upon or they overhear snide remarks being made about their affair. Sometimes the work group breaks into two factions, one supporting the affair and the other condemning it.

Unfair Access to Power

If a vertical hierarchical relationship exists, colleagues may feel threatened because a coworker has gained access to a person who has power.

Drop in Productivity and/or Work Quality

This decrease may involve not only the romantic couple, but also other employees who are indirectly involved or who waste time discussing the progress of the affair.

Disruptions of the Work Environment

Emotional explosions may occur when one or both partners are married to others and one of their spouses comes storming onto the work scene or into the supervisor's office.

Strained Relations or Work Conflicts .

These are particularly common when an affair ends.

POLICIES REGARDING OFFICE ROMANCES

Only a few organizations have specific written policies concerning romantic relationships at work. Those that do usually attempt to cope by one of the following mechanisms:

- Romances covered by sexual harassment policies.
- Employment of spouses prohibited.
- One person must resign or be terminated.
- Both may not work in same department.

PRACTICAL APPROACHES TO ADDRESSING WORKPLACE ROMANCES

1. There is no problem with performance or relationships with fellow workers. Both parties are single, and no organizational policy exists.

   Solution: Do nothing.

2. There is no problem with performance or relationships with fellow workers. The romance is an extramarital affair.

   Solution: Alert and advise. Often the parties think that they have kept the affair secret. State what you have heard and that employees are spending a lot of time talking about it. Admit that it is none of your business to interfere in their private lives, but as a friend you must urge them to give serious consideration to what they are getting into. If a policy prohibits on-the-job romances, warn them that they are treading on thin ice.

   When dealing with a clandestine relationship, expect the parties to vigorously deny that anything is going on. The best approach at that point is to avoid addressing the denials because everyone in the discussion knows the true nature of the affair.[3]

3. There is no problem with performance or relationships with fellow workers. Both parties are single, but a policy prohibits such activities.

   Solution: Counsel. Before you do anything, make certain that a written policy is really in effect. Often the message is conveyed verbally, not from rules but from an executive (eg, "Sally, you have got to do something about the relationship between Jim and Mary"). Review the policy carefully, then discuss it with the pair. Tell them what you will have to do if they persist in their activities.

4. There is a problem with productivity.

   Solution: Counsel. Use the same approach you would for employees who have substance abuse or other personal problems. Do not accuse them of having an affair, but simply show them how their performance has been slipping and that, while you have no intention of interfering in their personal relationship, they must return to their previous levels of performance.

   Most advisors recommend that this counseling be supportive rather than threatening. It is best done in three steps. First, discuss it with each person privately, and then with both of them together. If it is a vertical relationship, the major responsibility should rest with the higher-ranking person, and that person should be approached first.[1]

LEGAL PITFALLS

When one or both parties is fired or even transferred, a strong possibility exists that legal rebuttals may result. These actions are especially hazardous when only the woman is dismissed. If discharges and transfers are resorted to, they must be enforced equally between the male and female partners.[1]

REFERENCES

1. Westhoff LA. What to do about corporate romance. *Manage Rev.* 1986;75:50-55.
2. Warfield A. Coworker romances: impact in the work group and on career-oriented women. *Personnel.* 1987;64:22-35.
3. Mondy RW, Premeaux SR. People problems: the workplace affair. *Manage Solutions.* 1986;31:36-39.

27. Troubled Employees

Troubled employees are those who have any kind of personal problem that limits their ability to perform their jobs, such as family stress, alcohol or drug abuse, emotional disorders, or legal or financial difficulties. Health care employees are particularly vulnerable to substance abuse because they have stressful jobs and readily available access to controlled substances.[1] Supervisors provide an organization's first line of defense in dealing with troubled employees. Unfortunately, many supervisors adopt an avoidance strategy for handling such employees.[2]

TRANSIENT PROBLEMS

Many employees go through trying periods because of poor health, family conflicts, financial problems, or other crises. These episodes may be characterized by decreased productivity, tardiness, absenteeism, emotional outbursts, or irritability.

Over the short haul, only compassion and understanding are needed in these temporary situations. Tell these employees that you realize that they are going through a stressful situation, and ask how you can help. Better still, suggest specific ways that you can help (eg, modify their work schedules, revise target dates for special projects, or leave early on days when they have urgent outside responsibilities). If the condition persists, urge them to get professional help. Recommend your organization's Employee Assistance Program (EAP).

When employees are scheduled to undergo surgical or other special treatment or complex diagnostic tests, do not relate worst-case scenarios you have heard or express concern over their choice of physician or hospital. Help them to feel secure. Review with them company policy about sick leave, insurance, etc. Focus on the future (eg, "When you come back, then..."). When employees return after an illness, welcome them back and tell them they were missed. Avoid constantly asking them how they feel, but be prepared to listen to their concerns. Do not ask for details of operations or symptoms.

AIDS IN THE WORKPLACE

What should you do, if anything, when one of your employees tells you that he or she has AIDS or AIDS-related complex (ARC)? Opinions range from moralistic to practical on how to handle AIDS in the workplace.[3] Federal law requires that employees with AIDS be treated as medically disadvantaged persons. Like any other minority group, they are protected against discrimination.

A policy regarding AIDS should affirm the employer's concern for the health of employees with AIDS or ARC and a commitment to compassionate handling of these employees. A nondiscrimination practice in personnel selection, task assignment, training, promotion, and firing should be included.

Employees may not be concerned about AIDS until a coworker comes down with the disease or is simply rumored to have it.[3] With rare exception, coworkers must continue to work with infected employees or face the risk of dismissal.

Most organizations provide supervisors and employees with educational materials regarding AIDS, and medical benefits usually include the diagnosis and treatment.

The answer to the question posed at the beginning of this section is to treat that person like any other employee, keeping in mind that he or she has the same federally protected status against discrimination as a member of any other minority group.

DRUG AND ALCOHOL ABUSE

Drug and alcohol abuse should be viewed as illnesses and treated as such. The U.S. Federal Rehabilitation Act of 1973 protects workers who use alcohol and legal drugs as long as their usage does not interfere with job performance or cause a risk in safety standards.[4]

Policies

The first step in limiting the costs and liabilities of substance abuse is to develop a clear policy on drugs and alcohol. The second step is to communicate the policy to all employees.[1]

Policies must include a clear statement of the employer's rights and responsibilities when an employee's behavior or performance is unacceptable as a result of drug and alcohol abuse. It must also address the rights and responsibilities of employees.[4] Employee rights are those of privacy, confidentiality, and due process regarding disciplinary actions, availability of treatment, and any work accommodation during recovery phases. Employee responsibilities are to report for work in a sober, drug-free state and to refrain from imbibing alcoholic spirits or taking drugs that affect performance during working hours and on-site.

A policy should state management's willingness to commit resources to alleviate the problem, to ensure respect for employee's rights, and to abide by applicable federal, state, and local statutes and regulations.[4] Most employers recognize the importance of drug prevention programs and counseling and have made these services available. Some hospitals provide counseling within their facilities, while others, to ensure confidentiality, contract for these services elsewhere.

Typical Reactions of Supervisors

Most supervisors are not professional counselors or law enforcement officers. Their concern is noting changes in job performance, not sniffing breath. They are, however, responsible for their subordinates' performance and safety. All too often they practice enabling behaviors that actually help addicted employees to continue their downward slide. Inexperienced supervisors are likely to react as follows:

1. *They deny the problem's existence or importance.*
Most supervisors are reluctant to force an intervention even when it is needed to save an employee's career. Some supervisors are even reluctant to document unsatisfactory work performance.[5]
> "I do not see any users around here."
> "It is not really affecting their work."

2. *Their reasoning is faulty.*
They assume that people can control their addictions without outside help. They believe the employee's promises to change, or they attribute the deterioration of performance to other causes.
> "I would hit the bottle too, if I had to live with Joe's family situation."

3. They find excuses for their inaction.
"I am only his supervisor. I will let the chief nail him."
"How do you think that would make us look?"

4. They cover up the problem.
They achieve this by ignoring behavior, hiding mistakes, accepting or even providing excuses for the abusers, or doing the employee's work.

5. They accuse, criticize, or threaten.
"Bill, you have got to lay off the sauce."
"Laura, someone told me you snort crack cocaine. I am going to keep my eye on you."

6. They play doctor or lecture on the evils of drugs.
Unless managers are psychologists or professional counselors, they should not attempt to counsel the employee about substance abuse. Discussions should be limited to work performance and attendance and to recommendations for professional counseling.

7. They fail to recommend treatment.
Although supervisors may properly address the performance or attendance of the employee without making any accusations of substance abuse, they fail to express concern that some personal factor may be responsible for the dysfunctional performance and do not suggest that counseling may be appropriate. They may not be familiar with the available services and how these services can be obtained. They may even be guilty of making negative comments about the efficacy of the remedial programs that are offered.

8. They continue to put up with it.
The worst mistake of all for employers to make is to continue to put up with marginal performance, Monday morning absences, obvious signs of hangovers, long lunch breaks away from the premises, or other evidence of substance abuse. They may even cover for the person when he is absent or "under the weather."

The TTT Solutions

Tolerate
To tolerate the abuse of controlled substances is unfair to the abuser as well as to the organization. Toleration is an indication of either supervisory failure or the unwillingness of management to support supervisory actions. For example, a nurse in charge of an operating suite may fail to report a surgeon who reeks of alcohol, or the nurse may report the surgeon, but the adminis-

tration fails to take action because the surgeon brings many patients into the hospital.

Treat
Guiding employees to professional treatment is the best course.

Terminate
Termination is the quickest solution, but seldom the best. Employers have learned—or are learning—that it is not only more humane to provide therapy, but it is also cost effective. Employers have discovered that it is more expensive to replace employees than it is to retain them by providing the help they need. Termination is appropriate only when attempts at treatment have failed.

Training of Supervisors and Employees

Supervisors must understand the reasons behind the drug and alcohol policy and be able to respond effectively to situations that require intervention. Because of possible negative ramifications, both personal and legal, they should not attempt remedial counseling. Poor advice can damage working relationships, and supervisors invite legal complications if they offer inappropriate advice.[6]

Managers should receive special training in how their EAP (or alternative support program) functions, when and how to refer employees, and how to handle employees during and after treatment. Here are some topics frequently covered in such training programs[7]:

- Explanation of drug and alcohol abuse policy.
- Information about commonly abused drugs and drug paraphernalia.
- Early identification of, and intervention in, the problem.
- Monitoring changes in employee behavior.
- How management supports the supervisors in the enforcement of the policy.
- How to educate employees, including the explanation of dangers of drug abuse, the policies of the organization, and the available help.

The Intoxicated Employee

Acute intoxication on the job calls for immediate action. The safety of the intoxicated person, the people around him, and the service activities are all at stake. If the employee is disorderly, security officers must be summoned. When employees show poor coordination, have slurred speech, or display other signs that they cannot perform their duties, they should be seen by a physician if one is on staff. If they are sent home, safe transportation must be provided. Disciplinary actions vary from employer to employer, but in all instances the episode should be documented.

On-the-job Signs of Alcohol and Drug Addiction

1. Appearance and Symptoms
Shaking hands, bloodshot eyes, puffy eyelids, lack of attention to personal hygiene; cough, weight loss, headaches, chronic gastritis; excessive perspiration.

Note: Chronic alcoholics frequently take prescription drugs such as Valium because of pain or insomnia.

2. Absenteeism
Excessive sick days for vague ailments; frequent absences on Mondays, Fridays, days after paydays, or holidays; unauthorized absences.

3. At Work but Not at the Workstation
Frequent trips to washroom; late returns from breaks; falling asleep during meetings or elsewhere; long lunches, often off the worksite (alcohol); seen talking to strangers in parking lot (drugs); secretive phone calls (drugs).

4. Marginal or Decreased Job Performance
Alternating periods of high and low performance; taking longer to do less, increased overtime, missed deadlines; increased errors or lapses of memory; increased accidents or safety violations.

5. Poor Relationships With Coworkers
Overreaction to criticism; mood swings, irritable, argumentative, outbursts of anger, inappropriate tears or laughter; borrowing money; avoiding coworkers and friends, or changing associates.

6. Other
Disappearance of medical alcohol or drugs; wearing dark glasses indoors; blood stains on shirt sleeves (drugs).

Steps in Coping

1. Assess the Situation
Look for the signs previously listed. Ask yourself these questions:

- Was the person always like this, or is this new?
- Has there been a definite change in performance or behavior?

- How do the employee's coworkers feel about alcohol or drugs? If either is tolerated—even encouraged—you may have a more pervasive or refractory problem.
- Does this interfere with the person's duties? Is it affecting coworkers, customers, the reputation of the institution or the public?

2. Document All Instances of Declining Job Performance

Be specific. Record dates, times, places, nature of incidents, and any other important information. Base these incidents on documented or well-established minimal acceptable levels of work standards or behavioral policies.

3. Consult With Behavioral Expert

Get help in formulating a strategy that is compassionate, avoids blaming, confronts behavior, and forces a solution by the offending person.

4. Confront the Employee

Interviews should deal only with the performance and should be structured to strive for a goal of a positive change in behavior. Basically, you handle these confrontations the same way you would when interviewing any marginal employee. Supervisors are not qualified to treat diabetes, and they should not try to treat employees who have substance abuse problems.[2]

The tone of the interview should be one of support coupled with firmness. Describe how work is unsatisfactory, not what you suspect to be the cause. Do not voice suspicion of drug, alcohol, or psychiatric problems. Express concern, not sympathy. Stick to documented facts. Explain how performance has changed, and review acceptable performance levels.

Avoid red flag words like "careless," "stupid," "weakness," "should," "never," and "always," or statements that elicit defensiveness.

Give the employee a chance to respond. Listen attentively and patiently, and be prepared for resistance. Do not argue or make idle threats.[2] Be very reluctant to accept excuses (these individuals are masters at fabricating excuses).

If no explanation is offered, say, "I do not know what the problem is, Phil, and it is really none of my business. However, your performance is my concern, and something must be done about it."

Resist the temptation to give advice. Press your tongue against the roof of your mouth when you are tempted to say, "If I were you…" or "Here is what you should do…." There are several dangers in attempting to counsel: (1) the employee may no longer feel a need to seek the professional help that is really needed; (2) serving as counselor makes it difficult for you to change to disciplinarian later, should that become necessary; (3) the employee could resent your probing into personal affairs.

Be very specific as to what must be improved and how much improvement is needed. Warn as to what will happen if performance does not rebound. Reassure the employee that you are always willing to discuss performance. Specify a follow-up date to review the situation. Express confidence in the employee's ability to improve. For example:

> Supervisor: "Phil, your usual excellent performance has fallen off over the past month or so. Your reports used to be very prompt. However, the last three were late, and I had to return two of them because of significant errors. When I tried to review these with you, you accused me of nit-picking and stormed out of my office. Phil, several of your colleagues have complained about your mood swings. If you have a personal or medical problem, I would be happy to make arrangements for you to talk to someone who could help. Whatever you do, Phil, is up to you. But, I must insist that your performance return to what it used to be."
>
> Phil: "Are you accusing me of being a lush?"
>
> Supervisor: "No, I said that your performance has plummeted, and that you seemed to have a problem of some kind. I distinctly said that it was none of my business what that problem is."
>
> Phil: "Why don't you just go ahead and fire me?"
>
> Supervisor: "I don't want to fire you. I want to help you."
>
> Phil: "You suggested the EAP. Isn't that for druggies?"
>
> Supervisor: "No, the EAP is for anyone with a personal problem that is interfering with their ability to perform up to standard."
>
> Phil: "Everybody would know that I go there, right?"
>
> Supervisor: "Wrong, Phil. If you take advantage of our EAP right now, the referral will be completely confidential. However, if your performance does not improve, we may soon reach a point when you either get sacked or you get treatment. If that situation arises, the EAP counselor will have to keep me informed as to your progress."

After the meeting, document what was discussed and what agreement was reached. Give the employee a copy.

5. Provide Follow-up Information

If performance improves, meet again to provide feedback on progress, giving specific examples of improvement. Reiterate that you are confident that this new and improved level of performance will continue. Again, document the meeting and give the employee a copy.

If performance fails to improve, move from counseling to disciplinary interviews. Lay it on the line. State that the person's job is in jeopardy. One thing that people with alcohol or drug problems fear is loss of their jobs. Loss of job means loss of the wherewithal to support their habits. Do not make idle threats! For example:

> Supervisor: "Phil, your performance is still unsatisfactory. We are now at the crossroads. Either you get help with your problem or you lose your job. Which is it?"

Phil: "I guess I should get some help."
Supervisor: "Good, let me make an appointment with our EAP, OK?"

If the employee cooperates and gets treatment, continue your support and observation. Be patient to the extent of easing off on tight deadlines and extra work requirements, while still insisting that minimum documented standards of performance be met.

Never violate the person's trust. If he must take time off for therapy, simply announce at a staff meeting that he is on leave for personal reasons. When he returns, treat him like you would any employee returning from an illness. Alert your staff (eg, "Phil will be back Monday. I know you will all make him feel welcome and help him get back into the swing of things").

Expect occasional relapses. Give positive strokes for good work, while resisting the temptation to lighten the workload too much. Treat the person like you do other employees. Remember that a reasonable transition period may be required before performance reaches the desired level.

EMPLOYEE ASSISTANCE PROGRAMS

Progressive major employers have EAPs or some other means for providing counseling services to their employees. EAPs have broad applications. Although they are used most often for alcohol and drug problems, many EAPs extend their services to employees who have family, marital, or emotional problems. Financial advisors are sometimes available. Trust in the confidentiality of an EAP is the keystone of a successful program. Employees and supervisors must know that and have confidence in it. For that reason, EAPs are best located off premises. If they are in-house, the location should preclude the possibility of employees being recognized as clients. It is also critical to prevent an EAP from being looked on only as a means for employees to avoid disciplinary action.[1]

Supervisors should consult the EAP before making a referral. This allows the EAP to screen out people who would benefit more from some other modality. The advice of the EAP also helps to protect employers from future litigation.

If an employee calls the EAP based on a supervisor's informal suggestion, it is usually considered to be a self-referral, and the supervisor does not receive any feedback from the EAP. In the case of a formal supervisory referral, the employee may be required to contact the EAP for assessment or to face dismissal. However, no specifics are given out about the identified problem or the treatment regimen. The supervisor is told only that the employee has contacted the EAP and has agreed to a treatment plan. A second report is sent to the supervisor at the completion of treatment.

WORKAHOLICS

Most workaholics do not perceive themselves to be difficult people. However, people who must work with or for workaholics will tell you that these intense folks are not very easy to get along with.

Machlowitz,[8] who is a workaholic, has described workaholics for the most part in positive terms. She says that they are surprisingly happy doing what they love—work. They are energized rather than enervated by their work, which they perceive as a hobby. She also found that most employers are delighted to have some workaholics on their staffs. Some would like to get them cloned.

Machlowitz admits that their underlying pattern is obsessive-compulsive; their personality behavior pattern is type A—intense, energetic, and driven. They are addicted (to their job) like alcoholics, but their addiction is more of a virtue than a vice. They have strong self-doubts and secretly suspect that they are inadequate. They fear failure.[8]

Workaholics as bosses are busy but not always effective because they delegate poorly and tend to be demanding, expecting everyone to work as hard as they do, thus creating a pressure cooker atmosphere.[8] If you work for one, anticipate and respond to their sense of urgency. Find out exactly what is expected, make certain that you are adequately rewarded for what you do, and let your boss know when you are and are not available. If you fail to do this, you will get calls at all hours of the day and night, and be expected to be on call all the time. You may have to decide if working for such a person is worthwhile.[8]

Managers who supervise workaholics have their work cut out for them. Workaholics are not good team players and tend to be glory-grabbers. They need and expect attention to be paid to their exploits. They tend to compete rather than to collaborate.[8] Since workaholics enjoy what they do, changing their life-style is all but impossible. However, some changes can be achieved.

Provide direction in establishing a priority list of projects and time frames for their completion.[9] Meet frequently to see what the workaholics have accomplished. Get them to make daily plans including a block of time for each activity.[9] Specific times should be set for them to leave work and take breaks. Encourage them to take up noncompetitive sports or hobbies that can be shared with family or friends.[9] Do not try to force them into team efforts.

THE DOS AND DON'TS OF COPING WITH TROUBLED EMPLOYEES

Do

- Establish work standards for each position.
- Know the policies and procedures of your organization.

- Record the performance of these employees. The most common error is lack of documentation.[5]
- Deal with unacceptable performance as soon as you can prove it.
- Base counseling or disciplinary action on job performance.
- Be ready to cope with resistance.
- Get a commitment and monitor it. Be firm and persistent.
- Show concern for the person without expressing sympathy.
- Maintain confidentiality.

Don't

- Ignore a problem or delay action.
- Apologize to offender for acting.
- Lecture or moralize.
- Mention alcohol, drug, or psychiatric illness.
- Try to be a diagnostician or therapist.
- Cover for person.
- Buy phony excuses.
- Award performance ratings that have not been earned.
- Expect too little from employee or too much from yourself.
- Make idle threats.

REFERENCES

1. Bensinger PB, Fitzpatrick SB. Facing up to substance abuse. *Health Maintenance Q*. 1987;9:9-11.

2. Mazzoni J. A supervisor's role in workplace drug abuse. *Health Care Supervis*. 1990;8:35-39.

3. Ross JK III, Middlebrock BJ. AIDS policy in the workplace: will you be ready? *SAM Adv Manage J*. 1990;55:37-41.

4. Pace L, Smits SJ. Workplace substance abuse: a proactive approach. *Personnel J*. 1989;68:84-88.

5. Campbell D, Graham M. *Drugs and Alcohol in the Workplace: A Guide for Managers*. New York, NY: Facts on File Publishers; 1988.

6. Longenecker CO, Liverpool PR. An action plan for helping troubled employees. *Manage Solutions*. July 1988:22-27.

7. Balevic HJ. *Report on Drug Abuse in the Workplace*. Washington, DC: Library of the Drug Enforcement Administration; 1985.

8. Machlowitz M. *Workaholics: Living With Them, Working With Them*. Reading, Mass: Addison-Wesley Publishing Co; 1980.

9. Haas R. Strategies to cope with a cultural phenomenon—workaholism. *Supervis Manage.* 1991;36:6.

28. Interpersonal Skills for the Health Care Supervisor

UMMING IT ALL UP

The main thrust of this chapter is to review briefly the contents of this book. As you read each paragraph you will probably encounter some items that do not sound familiar. When you find these, turn back to the indicated chapter and review that item. Repetition is a key to learning.

Chapter 1: Let's Meet These Difficult People

Supervisors who deal effectively with people employ proactive as well as reactive skills. These combined skills include power communication, assertiveness, and stress resistance. These in turn require a high level of self-esteem, enthusiasm, optimism, and a caring attitude that reaches out not only to clients, but also to colleagues and those above and below them in the organization. These qualities are essential for coping with difficult people, particularly because the health care environment and the characteristics of these employees are so unique.

Chapter 2: Powerful Communication Skills

All too often, managers tell their staffers only what the managers think the employees need to know. Employees want a lot more! Current changes in the racial and cultural make-up of our work force demand extra effort to avoid communications barriers. Even more important is the circumvention of psychological barriers such as sarcasm, put-downs, and inflammatory messages. Articulation that vibrates with energy, courtesy, and empathy is so important. Listening is by far the most valuable of the communications skills. Good listeners tune into feelings as well as to content. Upward communication is encouraged by being receptive to suggestions and even criticism.

Chapter 3: Self-Esteem and Assertiveness

Effective managers walk the fine line between assertiveness and aggressiveness. Passivity spells disaster. Any nonassertive health care professional who seeks a leadership role should attend a seminar, find an audiotape, or get a book on the subjects of assertiveness and self-esteem. Only when one can honestly report that she conforms to the Assertive Bill of Rights should this person feel prepared to face those difficult people out there.

Chapter 4: Stress

Successful team-builders and change-masters are resistant to stress. Their ability to facilitate, support, and stimulate their associates minimizes the stress that they, the managers, cause. It protects their employees from internal and external stressors and prevents the development of, or alleviates the effects of, problem people. They provide a nice balance between task and people orientation.

Chapter 5: The Employee Selection Process

Many potential problems with employees can be avoided if job applicants are screened more carefully. Conducting successful interviews to determine competency includes thorough questioning of candidates and their references. Batteries of questions that address not only technical or professional qualifications, but also motivation, compatibility, manageability, stress resistance, and truthfulness are needed.

Chapter 6: Better Orientation and Training of New Employees

Taking the time to properly orient and train new hires pays handsome dividends. Today's workers want to know not only what they will do and how to do it, but also why their tasks are important. When procedures, rituals, values, ethics, and philosophy of the organization are discussed, behavioral variances are less likely to occur. Supervisors who clue new staffers into the supervisors' personal likes and dislikes are much less apt to have to take remedial measures later.

Chapter 7: Coaching to Prevent Personnel Problems

Day-to-day coaching that features flexible leadership styles and multidirectional communication is the strongest proactive measure to avert and control interpersonal conflicts and emotional upsets. Managers who isolate themselves from their troops are not aware of potential problems. By the time problems move into their offices these managers find themselves facing major difficulties, which are often irreversible or require lengthy remedial measures. A competent coach ensures high productivity and compliance with the unwritten Employee Bill of Rights when she wears the hats of trainer, facilitator, counselor, consultant, delegator, supporter, problem solver, coordinator, peace maker, enforcer, and disciplinarian. Good coaches develop effective recognition and reward systems. They have the ability to motivate without relying on monetary rewards or promotions. They excel at praising and can reprimand without destroying self-esteem.

Chapters 8 and 9: Counseling and Disciplining Difficult Employees

When the behavior of difficult employees goes beyond the boundaries of acceptable deportment, supervisors must counsel or discipline these people. Counseling and disciplining are educational processes; the goal is to correct the behavior, not to punish the employee. Supervisors must have the courage to get rid of those people whose performance or behavior remains unacceptable.

Chapter 10: Conflict Resolution and Confrontation

As soon as we move from proactive to reactive coping, we enter the arena of conflict and confrontation. A host of etiologic and precipitating factors are available, and stereotypic responses must be replaced by flexible strategies that fit individual situations and persons. Assertive confrontations are enhanced by using success imagery and rehearsals. Confronting angry employees, colleagues, and clients requires special skill. The person who speaks first controls the mood; the person who asks the most questions controls the direction; and the person who listens best controls the outcome—back to communication skills.

Chapter 11: Principles of Coping With Difficult People

Supervisors can handle difficult people best when they are not only cognizant of the policies, rules, and procedures of their organization, but can also explain the reason for each. The three critical mistakes made by managers who are faced with problems are: (1) avoiding or delaying action; (2) ascribing undesired behavior to bad attitudes; or (3) gunnysacking. While common sense is important in all problem solving and decision making, unless supported by learned coping skills, it will often be ineffective.

Chapter 12: Difficult or Just Different

To a degree, individual differences correlate with potential interpersonal problems. These differences can be racial, cultural, gender-based, social, or religious. Equally important are differences in temperaments, values, and goals. The more we understand these variances, the less difficulty we will have getting along with others. The first step in this direction is analyzing and classifying our own temperament and that of our principal annoyers.

Chapter 13: High-Tech Professionals

High-tech professionals, such as physicians, laboratory scientists, and technical specialists, pose a special challenge to managers who lack previous experience in the health care industry. For one thing, these specialists often have more loyalty to their professions than to their employers. As shortages in the supply of these people increase, retention problems become acute unless these "wild ducks" are handled expertly. This handling includes careful recruitment and selection of candidates, orientation of new hires, flexible leadership styles, effective recognition and reward strategies, and opportunities for continuing education. Prima donnas and nonconformists require special handling.

Chapter 14: Difficult People at Meetings

Performance at meetings tends to bring out the worst in people. Tempers flare and personal agendas challenge the chairs. People who are not usually difficult can become very obstreperous. Keys to coping include the careful selection of attendees (when possible), thorough preparation, assertive communication skills, and artful leadership. Supervisors must know how to handle the habitually late arrivers, intimidators, know-it-alls, arguers, motor-mouths, and the silent passive members. The spectrum of problem members includes the hecklers, the comics, the negativists, and the destroyers.

Chapter 15: Difficult Patients ·

Difficult people are often more difficult when they become patients. Even the most congenial folks can be complaining, demanding, angry, depressed, or inconsiderate when they are ill. Client service demands that caregivers make allowances for these behaviors, but this does not mean always giving into unreasonable demands. The skilled caregiver has, in addition to empathy and professional skill, the ability to respond appropriately to patients who are overly complaining, demanding, verbally abusive, or manipulative, or who refuse treatment.

Chapter 16: Difficult Bosses

When supervisors deal with subordinates they have the advantage of authority. In the case of difficult colleagues, the playing field is level. Hierarchical superiors who are hard to get along with present a more challenging situation. Individuals whose expertise is in great demand are in the driver's seat. They can be choosy about selecting an employer and immediate superior, or they can test the waters and wave goodbye. In most instances, getting along with one's boss involves showing loyalty, empathy, adjusting to personalities, and accepting the boss as she is. Some behavior modification is possible by reinforcing desired behavior by positive strokes. Special problem bosses require special measures. These superiors include the ones who have an intense affiliation need, the con artists, the over- or underdelegators, the laissez-faire leaders, the procrastinators, the unfair bosses, the ones who manage by crisis, the reverse end-runners, the dyed-in-the-wool bureaucrats, the tyrants, and the ones with alcohol or drug problems.

Chapter 17: The Underperformers

Today's leaders are faced with the demand for increased service quality and productivity, without increased costs. Major barriers to achieving these goals are employees who are not productive. Most underperformance is attributable to poor leadership. Only a small percentage of employees do not want to perform well. Employees must know what is expected of them, how to do their jobs, and why their work is important. They want periodic feedback on how well they are performing. Special kinds of underperformers include the bitter, passed-over ones, the slow or spurt workers, the perfectionists, and the time wasters. If the practical solutions to these problems are given a fair shake and do not produce the desired results, then transfer, demotion, or separation is appropriate.

Chapter 18: Employees Who Do Not Show Up

Absenteeism is a major flaw in American organizations. The health care industry is no exception. Both traditional and nontraditional measures have been used by CEOs to curtail unexcused absences. Employee attendance varies directly with the quality of their supervision. Supervisors have three major responsibilities: (1) to provide competent leadership; (2) to interpret, promulgate, and enforce policies pertaining to attendance; and (3) to counsel and discipline chronic offenders.

Chapter 19: People Who Resist Change and Avoid Risk

The rate of technological advances and organizational shuffling demands flexibility at all levels. People who stand in the way of progress and change will be swept aside. Supervisors must be change specialists, leading their troops into new and sometimes uncharted and riskier waters. Most teams have individuals who resist change, thus becoming another group of difficult people. Six proactive strategies help to prevent change problems. Specific advice is offered for coping with the people we labeled as spectators, nonparticipants, skeptics, resisters, and the ones who fear any kind of risk.

Chapter 20: Unethical People

Increasingly, supervisors are faced with ethical issues. The major issues must be resolved by committees or other persons in authority. We focus on the medical and nonmedical decisions that managers and their associates must cope with on a daily basis. Each of us must formulate our individual value systems while also enforcing the codes demanded by our organization. Proactive measures to deal with ethos include the careful selection of where we work and for whom. Since managers have a controlling responsibility, they must be alert to and respond to unethical behavior. Obviously they must model what they preach.

Chapter 21: Bad Attitudes and Pessimists

When managers talk about their problem employees, the term heard most often is "bad attitude." Unfortunately, this subjective word has little meaning unless it is followed by descriptions of behavior. A bad attitude can refer to anything from disloyalty to slothfulness. We explore the reasons for poor attitudes and follow that with practical coping methods.

Chapter 22: Complaints and Chronic Complainers

Complaints are beneficial; chronic complainers are not. For most supervisors, legitimate complaints from employees and clients represent a major source of service feedback—all too often the only one. Alert managers take complaints seriously, discuss them with their staff, and keep a record of them. We provide you with six essential moves in addressing individual complaints and include seven tips on handling salary controversies. Chronic complainers and whiners are stingers for all managers. These people have very low self-esteem and suffer from constant frustration. While complete cure is seldom possible, their behavior may be modified.

Chapter 23: People Who Have Annoying Habits

We all deal with individuals who do their work satisfactorily but who say or do things that are annoying. These things may be minor annoyances such as articulating a "ya' know" in every sentence, or these people may drive you up with wall by responding to your questions with tight-lipped silence. This group includes the know-it-alls, the super-sensitives, the moody ones, jealous coworkers, incessant talkers, those who try to dump on you or go over your head, and those whose appearance or conversation is unacceptable. Each of these requires special and specific handling. We also focus on dealing with staffers who are feuding on the job.

Chapter 24: Hostile People

In his book and tapes on coping skills, Bramson provides a classic chapter on three kinds of hostile people. He labels them Sherman Tanks, Exploders, and Snipers. Drawing heavily on Bramson's descriptions, we discuss these people after giving some general advice on dealing with hostility.

Chapter 25: Sexual Harassment

Sexual harassment has not shown any signs of abating. We clarify the different forms and manifestations of sexual harassment and describe how special policies must be formulated, broadcast, and implemented. Step-by-step investigation of complaints are detailed and advice is offered on how you should react to a sexual harasser when you are the target.

Chapter 26: Romances in the Workplace

Office romances often pose management conundrums for supervisors. Depending on the circumstances and the organization's policies, appropriate solutions are discussed and the supervisor's role in coping with these is explained.

Chapter 27: Troubled Employees

Among the least pleasant responsibilities that supervisors must face is dealing with subordinates who have personal problems that are affecting their work or that of their teammates. Among the specific topics discussed are those of AIDS, drug and alcohol abuse, and the role of employee assistance programs. Detailed suggestions, including recommended dialogues, are described with warnings on how not to ignore these emotional issues. Emphasized repeatedly is the importance of confining discussions to work performance and not probing into personal lives or accusing employees of substance abuse.

A SUPERVISOR'S SURVIVAL KIT

Today's health care supervisors are busier than ever trying to keep up with all the external and internal forces that are bearing down on them, making their work ever more complex and demanding. Most supervisors have not yet felt the full impact of the latest Joint Commission on the Accreditation of Healthcare Organizations (JCAHO) requirements, new laws such as the Americans With Disabilities Act (ADA), and new regulations such as the Clinical Laboratory Improvement Amendments (CLIA '88).

CEOs are introducing sweeping changes in their organizational culture. Restructuring, merging, downsizing, satellite facilities, point-of-care services, and expansion of outpatient services take place with ever-increasing speed.

The changing characteristics of our work force necessitate increased attention to cultural diversity. Top management is demanding that supervisors empower their employees and develop autonomous or semi-autonomous work teams, often without telling the supervisors how to do it. As operations are streamlined, supervisors find themselves deeply involved in cross-functional operational groups. Supervisors are expected to accomplish more with less, to improve quality, to reduce turnaround time, to dazzle customers with their service, and to keep morale high.

And wait—there's more! Competitors are springing up all around us. We have expanded physician clinics and office laboratories, free-standing surgicenters, and other outside enterprises. Lurking in the background are the unions, ever ready to capitalize on employee dissatisfaction and now encouraged by the new federal law that permits multiple unions to invade each hospital.

To meet these tremendous challenges, supervisors must fine-tune their interpersonal skills, especially their ability to cope with difficult people. The advice given in this book serves as an additional management tool for your "supervisor's survival kit." You may have skipped over some of the chapters. If so, please give them a second try. You will find some practical advice that you missed in your first reading. More importantly, when you encounter a difficult person, use the book as a reference and study the appropriate section before your next encounter with them. Such preparation is the secret to your supervisory success!

Index

Boss
difficult, 137-147
with alcohol problem, 145-146
bureaucratic, 144-145
chain of command, not following, 144
con artist, 142
dealing with, 140-147
with drug problem, 145-146
"hands-off" leader, 142
management-by-crisis, 143
more than one, working for,
146
with need to be liked, 141
procrastinator, 142-143
threatened by employee, 146
tyrant, 145
unfair, 143
loyalty to, 138-140
new, adaptation to, 141
relationship with, 138
resistance to change, 171
selection of, 138
unethical behavior of, 180-181
"Brag sheet," for stress resistance,
32
Brain, hemispheres of, informa-
tional processing, 103-104
"Broken record" technique, 23
Bureaucrat, as boss, 144-145
Burnout
self-analysis of, 27-28
symptoms of, 25-26
Business meetings. See Meetings

C

Chain of command, disregard of,
211
by boss, 144
Change
communication about, 168-169
empowerment of employee, 169-
170
nonparticipant and, 171

obstructionists, 171-174
patience with, 170
preventing problems of, 168-171
reassurance, to employees, 169-
170
resistance to, 167-172
by boss, 171
reasons for, 168
skeptic and, 171-172
spectator and, 171
validation of employee's feelings
with, 169-170
Characteristics, of difficult people, 1
Chronic absenteeism, dealing with,
164-165
Chronic complaints, 196-198
Civil Rights Act, employment discrimination, 37
Collaboration, in conflict confrontation, 85
Colleague, dishonesty/unethical
behavior, 181-183
Comic behavior, during business
meetings, 125
Committee, ethics, consultation
with, 168
Communication
anger, dealing with, 23-24
appearance, attentive, 9-10
auditory, 7
barriers to, 6-7
body language, 7
"broken record" technique, 23
as cause of conflict, 82
criticism, 12-14
feedback, 10
negative, 12-14
with high-tech professional, 116
of institutional change, 168-169
kinesthetic, 7-8
lines of, 6-5
neurolinguistic programming, 8
pause, 8-9
power, reduction of, 9
response, types of, 10-11
sexual harassment policy, 227

F

Facilitation, business meetings, 121-122
Favoritism, sexual harassment, 226
Fear, 30
Feedback, 10
    absence of, as cause of underperformance, 151
    employee orientation, 52
    negative, 12-14, 59
Feud, between individuals, dealing with, 211-213
Fighting, in conflict confrontation, 84
First impressions, of patient, 128
"Fogging," in response to difficult patient, 133-134

G

"Game playing," in dealing with employees, 97-100
Gossip, dealing with, 213
Governance, hospital middle management, 3
Graduate, recent, hiring of, 42
Grievance procedure, for sexual harassment complaint, 228
Guidelines, and ethics, 177-178
Guilt, 18-19, 30-31

H

Habit, irritating, individual with, 207-208
"Hands-off" leader, as boss, 142
Health care environment, 3
Health care institution
    changes in, 167
    ethics and, 176-178
Health care supervisor, interpersonal skills, 249-257
Heckling behavior, during business meetings, 125

Hemisphere, brain, information processing, 103-104
Hidden agenda, at business meetings, 126
High-tech professional
    applicant, 114
    characteristics of, 112-114
    communication with, 116
    compatibility issues, 111-117
    educational opportunities for, 116
    horizontal leadership, 115
    leadership style, 114-115
    nonconforming, 116-117
    orientation, 114
    performance feedback, 115-116
    reward system, 115-116
    training, 116
Hiring
    Age Discrimination in Employment Act, 37
    Americans With Disabilities Act, employment discrimination, 37
    application evaluation, 35-36
    Civil Rights Act, employment discrimination, 37
    compatibility, of prospective employee, 39
    discrimination in, 36-38
    Equal Employment Opportunities Act, employment discrimination, 37
    interview, 36
        questioning process, 38-41
    intuition in, 42-43
    manageability, of prospective employee, 40
    motivation, of prospective employee, 39
    probationary period, 43
    "reasonable accommodation" of employee, 37-38
    recent graduate, 42
    references, reliable, obtaining, 41-42
    résumé evaluation, 35-36